OSTEOPOROSIS DIET COOKBOOK FOR SENIORS

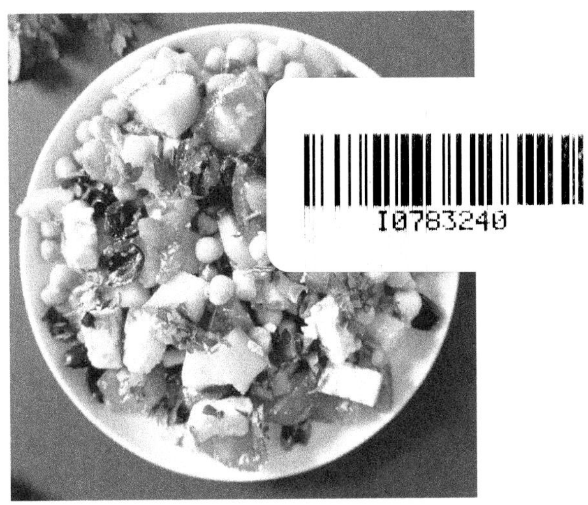

KEEP YOUR BONE STRONGER WITH DELICIOUS RECIPES AND EXERCISE

PATRICIA J PETERSON

Copyright ©2024 PATRICIA J PETERSON

All right reserved

No part of the book may be reproduced in any form or by any electronic or mechanic means, including information storage and retrieval systems, without the permission in writing from the publisher, except by a reviewer who may quote brief passage in a review.

The information in this book is true and complete to the best of our knowledge. All recommendations are made without guarantee on the part of the author or publisher. The author and publisher disclaim any liability in connection with the use of this information.

Table of Contents

CHAPTER ONE

1 INTRODUCTION TO OSTEOPOROSIS

Osteoporosis is a disorder in which bones deteriorate, making them more brittle and prone to fractures. Bone loss is known as the **"silent thief"** since it happens without any symptoms. Bones are living tissue composed of a hard outer shell and a spongy interior matrix that are constantly broken down **(resorption)** and regenerated **(formation)**. This process is known as bone remodeling, and it is necessary for the strength and health of bones throughout life.

The Basics of Bone Health

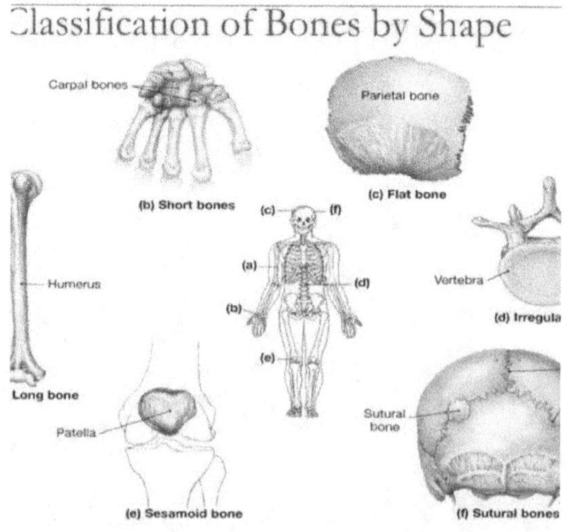

Bone density and quality are important indicators of overall bone health. Bone density, which measures how closely cells are packed together, peaks in early adulthood. After attaining maximal bone mass, the equilibrium of bone resorption and production may alter, resulting in bone loss over time. Bone quality, on the other hand, refers to the architecture, turnover, damage healing, and mineralization processes that occur inside the bone and contribute to its strength.

Factors influencing bone health:

Several variables can affect bone health, including:

- Genetics: Hereditary factors influence bone density and risk of osteoporosis.
- Nutritional Intake: Calcium and vitamin D are essential for healthy bone growth and maintenance. Magnesium, phosphorus, and vitamin K are additional necessary nutrients.
- Physical Activity: Weight-bearing and muscle-strengthening workouts help create and maintain bone density.
- Lifestyle Choices: Smoking and heavy alcohol usage can harm bone health.

- Hormonal Levels: Hormones, particularly estrogen in women, are important for bone density. Menopause promotes bone loss owing to a drop in estrogen levels.
- Medication and Medical Conditions: Certain drugs and medical conditions can have an influence on bone health, increasing the chance of developing osteoporosis.

Understanding osteoporosis.

Osteoporosis occurs when the production of new bone does not keep up with the loss of existing bone. This mismatch can result in porous, brittle bones that are prone to fracture, even under mild loads. Common fracture locations include the hip, spine, and wrist. These fractures can cause severe morbidity, worse quality of life, and, in the case of hip fractures, an increased risk of death.

The disorder is more common in older persons, particularly postmenopausal women, for the reasons listed above. However, osteoporosis can affect people of any age, gender, or ethnicity, emphasizing the importance of universal interventions for promoting bone health and preventing bone loss.

The Impact of Osteoporosis on Quality of Life

Osteoporosis is a disorder that slowly erodes the structural integrity of bones, leaving them vulnerable to fractures from modest falls or, in severe cases, basic daily activities. These fractures and the increasing weakening of bones have a substantial impact on people's quality of life in a variety of ways, including physical, emotional, and social.

Physical Impact

The most obvious effect of osteoporosis is an increased risk of fractures, especially in the hip, spine, and wrist. Hip fractures frequently necessitate surgery and can cause persistent disability, loss of independence, and the need for long-term care. Spinal fractures can cause persistent discomfort, limited mobility, and a stooped posture, limiting activities and contributing to a loss in physical health. The discomfort and physical restrictions associated with osteoporosis can lead to sedentary behavior, increasing the risk of additional bone loss and contributing to the development of other chronic illnesses.

Emotional and Psychological Impact

Individuals with osteoporosis may experience substantial psychological distress due to their worry of falling and incurring fractures. This dread may cause a decrease in activities and social connections, adding to feelings of isolation, despair, and anxiety. Visible postural changes, as well as the possible need for assistive equipment, can have an influence on self-esteem and body image, hurting mental health even more.

Social and Economic Impacts

Osteoporosis can have a significant social impact, influencing relationships, family dynamics, and involvement in community activities. The frequency of medical consultations, as well as the possibility of surgery and recovery, might strain personal relationships and restrict social involvement. The economic expenses of medical treatment, rehabilitation, and long-term care for osteoporosis-related fractures can be significant for both people and healthcare systems.

Impact on Independence and Daily Life

One of the most difficult elements of living with osteoporosis is loss of freedom. Daily chores and routines that were once taken for granted might become difficult or even impossible without support. Adapting to these changes can be upsetting and difficult, resulting in a worse quality of life.

Coping Strategies

Osteoporosis can be effectively managed with a mix of medical therapy, lifestyle adjustments, and support. Regular and proper exercise can assist improve balance, muscular strength, and bone health, lowering the risk of falls and fractures. Nutritional techniques for getting enough calcium and vitamin 0044 are also important. Individuals who get psychological assistance, such as therapy, support groups, or social networks, can better cope with the emotional issues of osteoporosis. Finally, education on fall prevention and home safety can help people keep their independence and quality of life.

Recognizing Symptoms and Diagnosing Osteoporosis

Osteoporosis is commonly referred to as the "silent disease" since it can proceed without symptoms until a fracture occurs. However, there are indications and risk factors that can suggest the existence of osteoporosis, and detecting them early can be critical for diagnosis and therapy. Understanding the diagnostic procedure for osteoporosis is also critical for implementing prompt therapies to control and minimize its effects.

Recognizing symptoms

Osteoporosis presents with no symptoms at first. As the illness advances, it may express itself in different ways, including:

- **Fractures:** These can result from modest falls or, in severe cases, from basic activities such as leaning over or coughing, with a focus on fractures in the hip, spine, and wrist.

- **Loss of Height:** Gradual loss of height or a stooped posture may indicate vertebral fractures and a decreasing spinal column caused by osteoporosis.

- **Chronic back pain**, which is caused by cracked or compressed vertebrae, is an early symptom of osteoporosis.

- **Noticeable Posture Changes:** A stooped posture or the appearance of a "dowager's hump" (a rounded upper back) may suggest spinal bone loss.

Risk Factors:

Certain factors can increase the chance of having osteoporosis, including:

- Age: The risk increases as you become older, particularly around 50.

- Sex: Women are more prone to develop osteoporosis, especially after menopause, due to reduced estrogen levels.

- A family history of osteoporosis or bone fractures may increase risk.

- Small, slender people are more vulnerable since they have less bone mass.

- Lifestyle Choices: Smoking, heavy alcohol intake, and sedentary behavior can all raise the risk.

- Dietary factors: Low calcium intake, vitamin D insufficiency, and eating problems can all weaken bones.

- Medical illnesses and therapies: Certain illnesses and drugs, particularly glucocorticoids and cancer therapies, can have an impact on bone health.

Diagnosing osteoporosis.

The primary method for diagnosing osteoporosis **is bone mineral density (BMD) testing**, which is commonly performed using **dual-energy x-ray absorptiometry.** This non-invasive test determines the density of bone minerals (calcium) in particular parts of the skeleton, often the hip and spine, and compares the findings to average levels for a young, healthy person (T-score).

- T-score: A score of -1.0 or above is deemed normal. A score of -1.0 to -2.5 shows poor bone mass (osteopenia), whereas -2.5 or below suggests osteoporosis.
- Z-score: Sometimes used, particularly in younger people, to compare bone density to what is predicted for someone of the same age, gender, weight, and ethnic or racial background.

Additional tests may be performed to rule out other problems or uncover potential causes of osteoporosis, such as blood and urine testing to detect underlying disorders or vitamin deficiencies that may impair bone health.

Micronutrient Deficiency and Its Role in Osteoporosis

Osteoporosis is a disorder marked by weakening bones and an increased risk of fracture. While calcium and vitamin D are well known for their important functions in bone health, additional micronutrients are also required to maintain bone density and prevent osteoporosis. These vitamin deficiencies can play a key role in the development and progression of osteoporosis.

Essential Micronutrients for Bone Health.

Calcium: Calcium is the basic building block of bone tissue, and its role in bone health is critical. Calcium insufficiency can cause reduced bone density, fragility, and an increased risk of fractures.

- **Vitamin D**: Vitamin D is required for calcium absorption in the stomach, and a lack of it can lead to less calcium available for bone development and repair. This can cause brittle bones and a higher risk of osteoporosis and fractures.

- **Magnesium**: Helps convert vitamin D into an active form, which influences calcium metabolism and bone health. Magnesium shortage can affect the mineral content of bones, compromising their form and function.

- **Vitamin K** is important for the alteration of bone matrix proteins and aids in the binding of calcium to the bone matrix. Inadequate vitamin K levels can contribute to poor bone quality and strength.

- **Phosphorus** works in tandem with calcium to strengthen bones and teeth. Proper bone mineralization requires a balance of calcium and phosphorus.

- **Zinc** is required for bone tissue regeneration and mineralization; a zinc shortage can affect bone development and healing.

- **Copper** is involved in the synthesis of collagen for bone and connective tissue, and it works along with zinc to preserve bone strength.

The impact of micronutrient deficiencies on osteoporosis

Micronutrient deficits can have a significant influence on bone health, leading to the initiation and progression of osteoporosis in various ways.

- Impaired Bone Growth and Development: A lack of vital nutrients during critical phases of growth might result in insufficient bone mass buildup, increasing the risk of osteoporosis later in life.

- Decreased Bone Density: A lack of key micronutrients can slow down bone remodeling, resulting in lower bone density and more fragility.

- Increased Bone Loss: Certain micronutrient shortages can increase bone resorption while decreasing bone production, hastening bone loss and leading to osteoporosis.

Addressing Micronutrient Deficits

To reduce the risk of osteoporosis, it is critical to address any potential vitamin deficiencies. This involves:

- Balanced Diet: Eating a range of foods high in critical nutrients, such as dairy products, leafy green vegetables, fatty fish, nuts, and seeds, will help keep micronutrient levels stable.

- Supplementation: In circumstances when food intake is insufficient, such as vitamin D during the winter months or in those with special dietary limitations, supplementation may be required.

- Regular Screening: Periodic medical exams can help detect micronutrient deficiencies early on, allowing for appropriate action.

CHAPTER TWO

2   BONE HEALTH

Bone remodeling is an ongoing process that involves the breakdown of old bone tissue and the development of new bone tissue. This dynamic mechanism enables bones to respond to stress, mend small injury, and maintain calcium homeostasis in the body. Understanding the basic basis of bone remodeling is critical for understanding how osteoporosis occurs and how it may be controlled or cured.

Bone Structure and Composition

Bones are complicated organs composed of several tissues, including osseous (bone) tissue, marrow, blood vessels, and nerves. Osseous tissue is made up of two layers: cortical bone, which is solid on the outside, and trabecular bone, which is porous. Bone's structure is designed to offer strength and flexibility, and its cells play key functions in its maintenance and function:

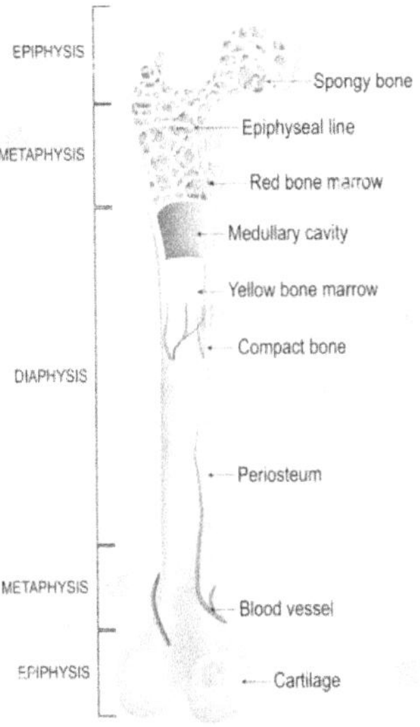

Osteoblasts are the cells responsible for bone production. They produce and exude collagen matrix and other proteins that mineralize to form new bone.

Osteoclasts are responsible for bone resorption; they break down bone tissue and release minerals like calcium back into the circulation.

Osteocytes are mature bone cells formed from osteoblasts that maintain bone tissue and control osteoblast and osteoclast activity.

Bone Remodeling

Bone remodeling happens in a well-organized cycle with various stages:

Activation: Pre-osteoclasts are drawn to remodeling areas.

Osteoclasts cling to the bone surface, creating an acidic environment that dissolves mineral content and digests the organic matrix, resulting in a resorption pit.

Reversal: Osteoclasts commit apoptosis (programmed cell death), while mononuclear cells prepare the location for future bone production.

Osteoblasts form new bone matrix in the resorption pit. This matrix then mineralizes, forming new bone.

This remodeling cycle is influenced by systemic hormones including parathyroid hormone (PTH), vitamin D, and calcitonin, as well as local variables like cytokines and growth factors.

Imbalanced bone remodeling and osteoporosis

Osteoporosis develops when there is an imbalance in the bone remodeling process, with bone resorption exceeding bone creation. Several variables may lead to this imbalance:

- Aging: As we age, the rate of bone resorption by osteoclasts increases, while bone synthesis by osteoblasts decreases, resulting in a net loss of bone mass.

- Hormonal Changes: In women, menopause causes a large fall in estrogen levels, which accelerates bone loss. In males, decreased testosterone levels with age can have a similar impact.
- Nutritional Deficiencies: A lack of calcium and vitamin D can reduce bone production and promote bone resorption, respectively.
- Lifestyle Factors: A sedentary lifestyle, heavy alcohol intake, and smoking can all lead to abnormal bone remodeling.

Factors that promotes bone loss

A variety of genetic, nutritional, lifestyle, and hormonal variables all have an impact on bone health. While bone loss is a normal part of aging, some illnesses and activities can hasten the process, raising the risk of osteoporosis and fractures. Understanding these characteristics is critical for designing ways to reduce bone loss and keep bones strong and healthy throughout life.

1. Hormone Imbalances

- **Estrogen and testosterone:** These sex hormones are essential for bone health. Women endure a fast period of bone loss in the first few years after menopause when estrogen levels fall. Men's testosterone levels gradually fall as they age, contributing to bone loss.

- **Thyroid hormones:** Excess thyroid hormone, whether caused by hyperthyroidism or over-replacement with thyroid hormone medicines, can cause greater bone loss.

- **Parathyroid Hormone:** Hyperparathyroidism, a disorder in which the parathyroid glands produce too much parathyroid hormone, can cause excessive calcium release from bones, weakening them.

2. Nutritional deficiencies.

- **Calcium and Vitamin D Deficiency:** One of the most important dietary variables contributing to bone loss is insufficient calcium and vitamin D consumption. Calcium is an essential component of bone, and vitamin D promotes calcium absorption and bone health.

- **Other Nutrients:** Calcium, magnesium, vitamin K, and phosphorus deficiencies can all have an impact on bone density.

3. **Lifestyle Factors.**

- **Physical inactivity:** Lack of weight-bearing and muscle-strengthening workouts might result in weaker bones. Exercise promotes bone growth and boosts bone density.

- **Smoking:** Tobacco usage has been related to lower bone density. Smoking has an effect on calcium absorption and estrogen levels, both of which are necessary for bone health.

- **Excessive alcohol** use can disrupt vitamin D metabolism, calcium balance, and hormone levels, all of which are necessary for healthy bones.

- **Caffeine:** Excess caffeine consumption may have a deleterious influence on bone health by interfering with calcium absorption.

4. **Medications**

Some drugs, such as:

- **Glucocorticoids:** Used to treat illnesses such as asthma and rheumatoid arthritis, they can reduce bone growth while increasing bone resorption.

- **Proton Pump Inhibitors (PPI):** Long-term use of PPIs may limit calcium absorption, potentially resulting in weaker bones.

- **Antiseizure drugs**: Some drugs used to treat seizures might cause bone loss.

5. Medical conditions.

Several chronic medical problems can harm bone health, including:

- **Rheumatoid Arthritis (RA):** Chronic inflammation caused by RA can reduce bone density.
- **Chronic kidney disease** can impair the body's capacity to absorb calcium and convert vitamin D to an active form.
- **Eating Disorders:** Conditions such as anorexia nervosa can result in malnutrition and bone loss.

6. Genetic Factors.

- **Family History**: Having a family history of osteoporosis or bone fractures enhances the chance of having the condition.

Bone density

Bone density, or bone mineral density (BMD), is an important indication of bone health and strength. It refers to the quantity of bone mineral in bone tissue, which indicates how thick and robust the bones are. The higher the bone density, the stronger the bones, reducing the chance of fractures. Bone density is an important element in detecting osteoporosis and determining fracture risk.

Importance of Bone Density

Bone density is important for various reasons.

- **Fracture Risk:** Lower bone density is linked to an increased risk of fractures, notably in the hip, spine, and wrist, which are all impacted by osteoporosis.
- **Osteoporosis** is diagnosed via bone density measures. A lower than normal bone density means that the bones are weaker and more likely to fracture.
- **Monitoring Bone Health**: Bone density examinations can track bone health over time, evaluating the efficacy of osteoporosis therapy or other bone density-related diseases.

Factors influencing bone density

Several variables can affect bone density, including:

Age: Bone density peaks in early adulthood and gradually diminishes with age.

- **Gender:** Women tend to have lower bone density than males and lose bone mass more quickly as they age, particularly after menopause.

- **Race & Ethnicity:** Certain populations, such as Asian and Caucasian women, are more likely to acquire osteoporosis.

- **Family History:** Genetics have an important impact in bone density.

- **Nutrition:** Getting enough calcium and vitamin D is vital for building and maintaining bone density.

- **Physical Activity:** Weight-bearing workouts assist to build and maintain bone density.

- **Lifestyle Choices:** Smoking and heavy alcohol intake can reduce bone density.

- **Medical Conditions and drugs:** Some conditions and drugs can reduce bone density.

Measuring bone density.

- **Dual-Energy X-ray Absorptiometry (DEXA or DXA)** scans are the most regularly used method for measuring bone density. This test is non-invasive, rapid, and the most accurate way to detect osteoporosis. It analyzes bone density at the hip and spine and returns a score that compares the measured bone density to the typical bone density of a healthy young adult (T-score) and persons of the same age, gender, and race (Z-score).

- **T-score:** The amount of bone you have compared to a young adult of the same gender at maximal bone mass. A T-score of -1.0 or higher is considered normal; -1.0 to -2.5 suggests poor bone mass (osteopenia), while -2.5 or lower implies osteoporosis.

- **Z-score:** Less typically used, but important if you suffer bone loss at an early age. It compares your bone density to the usual range for your age, gender, and size.

Managing and enhancing bone density

Improving and maintaining bone density requires a diverse strategy.

- **Diet**: A diet high in calcium and vitamin D is essential for bone health.

- **Exercise**: Regular weight-bearing and muscle-strengthening workouts can help increase bone density.

- **Lifestyle Changes:** Quitting smoking and reducing alcohol use are essential for preserving bone density.

- **Drugs:** For those who have osteoporosis or are at high risk of fractures, drugs can help enhance bone density and lower the risk of fractures.

Bone and Aging

As we age, our bones alter significantly, affecting their strength, density, and general health. Understanding the link between bone and aging is critical for preserving bone health and lowering the risk of osteoporosis and fracture.

Natural Bone Aging

- **Peak Bone mass achieves** its highest density and strength (peak bone mass) during the late 20s and early 30s. After this stage, bone remodeling continues, but the balance swings to more bone resorption than formation.

- **Bone Loss with Age**: Beginning in our 40s and 50s, the process of bone loss increases, particularly in women after menopause, due to a decrease in estrogen, a hormone required for bone density preservation. Men's testosterone levels gradually drop, which might impair bone density, but at a slower pace and later in life.

Factors Contributing to Bone Loss in Aging

- **Hormonal Changes:** Reduced estrogen and testosterone levels have a major impact on the pace of bone remodeling, resulting in an increase in bone resorption rather than creation.

- **Calcium and Vitamin D Absorption**: The body's capacity to absorb calcium and vitamin D, which are essential for bone health, declines with age. This might result in a deficit unless food intake is corrected or supplements are used.

- **Physical inactivity:** As people age, their physical activity levels may fall, lessening the mechanical stress on bones that encourages bone growth.

- **Chronic diseases and pharmaceuticals:** As people get older, the frequency of chronic diseases and the usage of medications that can lower bone density, such as glucocorticoids, rise.

Impact of Aging on Bones

- Increased Fracture Risk: The combination of lower bone density and an increased chance of falling raise the risk of fractures in older persons.

- Osteoporosis: As people become older, osteoporosis becomes increasingly frequent, especially among postmenopausal women, increasing their risk of fractures.

- Bone structure changes: Bones may grow thinner and more fragile. Bone microarchitecture deteriorates, making bones weaker and more prone to fractures.

Strategies to Mitigate the Aging Effects on Bones

- **Nutrition:** A sufficient supply of calcium and vitamin D is essential. Dairy, leafy green vegetables, seafood, and fortified foods should all be included in your diet. Supplements may be required depending on individual needs and medical recommendations.

- **Exercise:** Regular weight-bearing and muscle-strengthening workouts can aid to maintain bone density. Walking, dancing, yoga, and resistance training are all useful.

- **Lifestyle Changes:** Quitting smoking and reducing alcohol use are crucial for bone health. Maintaining a healthy weight without extreme dieting is also important for preventing bone loss.

- **Fall Prevention:** Lowering the risk of falling is critical for preventing fractures. This involves creating safe home surroundings, employing assistive equipment as needed, and doing balance and strength exercises.

- **Bone Density Screening:** Regular tests can diagnose osteoporosis early, allowing for prompt treatment. Medications may be provided to prevent additional bone loss and lower the risk of fractures.

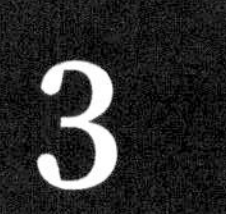

CHAPTER THREE

FRACTURE AND FALL

Fracture

A fracture, sometimes referred to as a bone fracture, happens when there is a disruption or fissure in the integrity of the bone. This can arise from a multitude of factors, including physical injury, excessive strain, and medical conditions that diminish bone strength, such as osteoporosis. Comprehending the intricacies of fractures is crucial for preventing, efficiently treating, and rehabilitating them.

Classification of Fractures

The severity of fractures can significantly differ based on the magnitude and orientation of the trauma, as well as the general condition of the damaged bone.

Typical categories comprise:

- A simple (closed) fracture occurs when the bone breaks but does not penetrate the skin.
- A compound (open) fracture occurs when the shattered bone penetrates through the skin, which heightens the likelihood of infection.

- A stress fracture is a little fissure in the bone caused by excessive usage or repetitive motion.
- A compression fracture commonly develops in the spine as a result of osteoporosis, causing the bone to collapse.
- Greenstick Fracture: Incomplete fractures that bend (frequent in youngsters whose bones are still pliable).

Causes and Risk Factors

- Trauma: Sudden hits or accidents are typical causes, including falls, sports injuries, and vehicle accidents.
- Osteoporosis: This disorder weakens bones, making them more prone to breakage from slight stress.
- Overuse: Repetitive actions can tire muscles and impose too much stress on the bone, leading to stress fractures.
- Cancer and Other illnesses: Certain malignancies and metabolic illnesses can weaken bones, increasing fracture risk.

Symptoms

Common symptoms of fractures include:

Intense discomfort at the location of the fracture, which may exacerbate with movement

- Swelling, bruising, or bleeding
- Visible malformation or misalignment of the limb
- Inability to exert weight on the afflicted area
- Loss of function in the damaged area

Diagnosis Diagnosis often requires a physical examination and imaging procedures such as X-rays to view the fracture. CT scans, MRI, or bone scans may be necessary for more complicated fractures or to monitor bone health.

Treatment

- Treatment varies on the fracture type, location, and severity. It seeks to straighten the bone, guarantee adequate healing, and restore function. Common treatments include:
- Casting or Bracing: To immobilize the bone and allow it to recover appropriately.
- Traction: Gently extending the muscles and tendons around the bone to align it.
- Surgery: In circumstances when bones cannot be straightened by non-invasive means, surgical solutions including metal rods, screws, or plates may be indicated.
- Physical Therapy: Essential for restoring strength and mobility in the damaged area following the first healing phase.

Prevention of fracture

Preventive interventions focus on lowering the risk factors for fractures:

- **Maintaining Strong Bones**: A diet rich in calcium and vitamin D, together with frequent exercise, especially weight-bearing and strength-training exercises, improves bone health.
- **Preventing Falls**: Especially in older persons, by reducing home dangers, enhancing lighting, and employing assistive equipment if needed.
- **Protection Gear**: Using adequate protection gear for sports and recreational activities.

Falls

Falls are situations that result in a person coming to rest accidently on the ground or floor or other lower level. While falls may occur at any age, they are particularly relevant in older persons because to the higher risk of serious damage, including fractures, brain injuries, and increased morbidity. Understanding the causes of falls and applying preventive measures is vital for preserving health and independence, especially as we age.

Causes of Falls Falls can come from a complex interaction of causes, commonly divided into intrinsic (individual) and extrinsic (environmental) components:

- **Intrinsic Factors**: Include age-related changes in balance and gait, diminished muscular strength, impaired vision, chronic diseases (such as arthritis, heart disease, or neurological problems), and adverse effects from drugs.
- **Extrinsic Factors**: Involve risks in the living environment, such as slippery flooring, insufficient lighting, congested paths, and improper footwear or assistance equipment.

Impact of Falls

The repercussions of falls extend beyond physical injury. They can lead to a fear of falling again, resulting in lower activity levels, social isolation, loss of independence, and psychological consequences including despair and anxiety.

Fall Prevention Strategies

Preventing falls entails addressing the numerous internal and extrinsic variables that contribute to the risk. Here are essential strategies:

- **Exercise and Physical Activity**: Engaging in regular exercise, particularly activities that promote balance, flexibility, and muscular strength, such as tai chi, yoga, and strength training, can greatly lower the risk of falls by increasing physical function.

- **Medication Management**: Regular assessments of medicines with a healthcare professional can detect and alter any drugs that may contribute to dizziness or instability.

- **Vision and Hearing Checks:** Regular exams help ensure that visual and hearing problems, which may increase the risk of falls, are effectively handled.

- **Home Safety Assessments**: Modifying the living environment to remove tripping hazards, enhance lighting, add grab bars in restrooms, and provide safe stairways and handrails can drastically lower the chance of falls.

- **Proper Nutrition and Hydration**: Adequate diet improves general health and energy levels, while regular water is crucial to prevent dizziness and balance concerns.

- **Education and Awareness**: Being aware about the risk factors and preventive methods for falls can empower individuals to take proactive efforts toward their safety.

Creating a Fall-Prevention Plan

A comprehensive fall-prevention strategy entails cooperating with healthcare practitioners, family members, and caregivers to analyze risk factors and implement appropriate solutions suited to the individual's requirements. This could involve a combination of fitness programs, home changes, medical interventions, and educational activities to establish a safe environment and promote healthy aging.

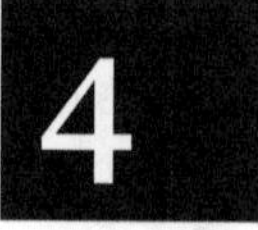 THE ROLE OF NUTRITION IN BONE HEALTH

Nutrition is critical for long-term bone health. Adequate consumption of particular nutrients is critical for forming strong bones and maintaining bone density and strength as we age.

Nutritional Foundations for Strong Bones

Building and keeping healthy bones is an important part of overall health that necessitates a consistent intake of key nutrients throughout one's life. Proper nutrition supplies the building blocks for bone production, aids in the prevention of bone loss caused by aging and lifestyle factors, and dramatically lowers the risk of osteoporosis and related fractures. Here, we look at the essential dietary components that contribute to bone health.

Essential dietary components

1. **Calcium** is essential for bone strength and density. It serves as the primary building block. It also aids in muscle function, neuron communication, and blood coagulation.

- Calcium-rich foods include dairy products (milk, cheese, yogurt), fortified plant-based drinks, leafy green vegetables (broccoli, kale), and fish with edible bones.

- The recommended daily consumption varies according to age, gender, and life stage, with higher requirements during adolescence, pregnancy, breastfeeding, and postmenopause.

2. **Vitamin D** has a crucial role in calcium absorption in the stomach, ensuring optimal serum calcium and phosphate levels for proper bone mineralization.

- **Vitamin D is naturally found** in the sun, but it may also be obtained from fatty fish, egg yolks, fortified milk, and supplements.

- **Recommended Intake:** Meeting vitamin D requirements through diet alone can be difficult, especially in areas with minimal sunshine exposure, hence supplementation is frequently required.

3. **Phosphorus:** Key to Bone Mineralization Phosphorus, in the form of phosphate, is essential for bone construction, energy storage, and transport throughout the body.

- **Sources:** A wide range of foods, including dairy products, meat, fish, poultry, nuts, seeds, and whole grains.
- **Balance with Calcium:** To achieve optimal bone health, the diet should have a suitable balance of phosphorus and calcium.

4. **Magnesium** as a Bone Quality Enhancer: Magnesium promotes bone structure and activates vitamin D. It also participates in about 300 enzymatic processes, including those necessary for energy generation and DNA synthesis.

- Green green vegetables, nuts, seeds, whole grains, and legumes are high in magnesium.
- **Recommended Intake:** Adequate magnesium intake is necessary for bone health and general metabolic function.

5. **Vitamin K**: A Matrix Modifier. Vitamin K is required for the formation of osteocalcin, a protein that binds calcium to the bone matrix, increasing bone strength and lowering fracture risk.

- **Sources:** Leafy green foods including kale, spinach, and Brussels sprouts are abundant in vitamin K. Fermented foods, such as cheese and natto (fermented soybeans), contain substantial quantities.

- **Recommended Intake**: Including a range of vitamin K-rich foods in your diet benefits both bone health and blood coagulation processes.

6. **Protein** is essential for bone health since it forms the bone matrix and aids in tissue repair and maintenance.

- Lean meats, poultry, fish, dairy products, legumes, and nuts are all good sources of protein.
- **Balance:** Protein should be consumed in moderation with other nutrients, since excessive intake, particularly from animal sources, can have a detrimental impact on bone health.

7. Additional micronutrients: Trace Elements of Bone Metabolism

- Zinc, Copper, Boron: These trace elements aid in collagen production and bone metabolism, hence promoting bone development and repair.
- **Sources:** A diversified diet that includes fruits, vegetables, nuts, seeds, meats, and whole grains usually offers enough levels of these micronutrients.

Super foods for Osteoporosis Prevention and Management

Incorporating particular items into your diet can help prevent and manage osteoporosis. These "superfoods" provide critical minerals such as calcium, vitamin D, magnesium, vitamin K, phosphorus, and omega-3 fatty acids, all of which are necessary for bone density and general bone health. Here's a look at some of these superfoods and how they might help prevent or treat osteoporosis.

1. **Dairy Products:** High in calcium and fortified with vitamin D, dairy products such as milk, yogurt, and cheese are beneficial for bone health.

- Tip: Choose low-fat choices to optimize advantages while avoiding extra saturated fats in your diet.

2. **Leafy Green Vegetables:** Kale, collard greens, spinach, and broccoli are high in calcium, magnesium, and vitamin K, all of which promote bone health.

- Tip: Include a mix of these veggies in your diet to benefit from a diverse range of antioxidants and other health-boosting elements.

3. **Fatty Fish Benefits:** Salmon, mackerel, tuna, and sardines have significant levels of omega-3 fatty acids and are natural sources of vitamin D.

- Tip: Aim for two servings of fatty fish each week to promote bone and cardiovascular health.

4. **Nuts and Seeds:** Almonds, chia seeds, flaxseeds, and walnuts contain calcium, magnesium, and omega-3 fatty acids, making them beneficial for bone health.

- Sprinkle them over salads, yogurts, or smoothies for an added nutritious boost.

5. **Fortified Foods Benefits:** Calcium and vitamin D fortified foods and beverages can assist satisfy daily requirements, especially for lactose intolerant individuals or those who struggle to obtain these nutrients from other sources.

- Tip: Look for fortified plant milks, orange juice, cereals, and bread as easy supplies of these essential nutrients.

6. **Soy Products Benefits:** Soybeans, tofu, tempeh, and soy milk include calcium and protein. They also contain isoflavones, which are related to better bone health.

- Tip: To maximum health advantages, use minimally processed soy products.

7. **Eggs Benefits:** Eggs naturally contain vitamin D, which is essential for calcium absorption and bone health.

- Tip: While the yolk contains vitamin D, eating the whole egg delivers other nutrients such as protein and vitamin B12.

8. **Prunes:** High in antioxidants, vitamin K, and manganese, prunes have been linked to reduced bone loss.

- Tip: Eat them as a snack or mix them into cereals and baked goods for a nutritional boost.

9. **Benefits of Whole Grains:** Magnesium, found in oats and quinoa, is crucial for bone building.

- Tip: Replace refined grains with whole grains to improve your diet's overall nutritional profile.

Foods to Limit or Avoid

Caffeine is connected with osteoporosis due to its interference with calcium absorption and its direct influence on bone. Caffeine intake has been connected with a loss in bone mass and an increase in fracture risk. High intake (6 or more cups a day) is regarded to be the threshold at which this harmful effect is most likely to occur. Limiting caffeine is helpful for both short-term and long-term bone health, as it helps to create and maintain optimal bone density throughout the key growing years and prevent bone loss in the elderly.

Alcohol also promotes the body to eliminate calcium in the urine and interferes with the absorption of calcium. It also has little nutritional benefit in terms of vitamins and minerals and is commonly eaten instead of other drinks that would offer calcium to the diet, such as milk or calcium-fortified drinks. Consider cutting out alcohol totally to boost your bone health.

High-sodium meals are a clear no-no in the daily nutrition of an osteoporosis sufferer. Sodium causes the body to lose calcium in the urine and interferes with absorption of calcium in the body. Carbonated soft drinks include phosphoric acid, which some studies have indicated is connected with an increase in calcium excretion in the urine. They also include caffeine, which has similarly been proven to promote the loss of calcium and interfere with calcium absorption. So, by opting to consume carbonated soft drinks rather than a glass of milk, we are losing out on a critical calcium-rich meal that we need to take frequently for the health of our bones.

High acid preservatives in fizzy drinks can damage the protective covering on the teeth and bones. These acids are not naturally occurring and the body does not have the capacity to neutralize them, therefore the body utilizes the reserves of calcium in the teeth and bones. High sugar and caffeine content in fizzy drinks can contribute to an increase in loss of calcium in the bones, especially at risk are women who are postmenopause. A research indicated that women who consumed more than 1 cola drink a day had a substantially increased risk of hip fractures from osteoporosis. The alternative of diet fizzy drinks is not suggested since these also have detrimental effects on the calcium reserves in the body and have no nutritional advantages.

White bread has a high glycemic index. The body reacts to it in a similar way to sugar and thus pulls calcium from the bones to digest it. This, in turn, can raise the risk of hip fractures. A research indicated that women who ate 2 pieces of white bread a day had a substantially increased risk of osteoporosis hip fractures. Substitute white bread for full grain or mixes such as rye or pita.

Processed foods have the potential to be harmful to the bones. They frequently include a high phosphorus concentration and low calcium content, which might be dangerous. The preparation of the meals may also produce a rise in the acids supplied as preservatives. This, in turn, might cause an increase in the loss of calcium in the bones. High salt concentration in processed meals promotes an accelerated loss of calcium in the bones, which can raise the risk of osteoporosis and fractures. Salt might also make you lose more calcium when you go to the bathroom. This is because the body requires calcium to assist the kidneys get rid of the salt. High sugar level can also be harmful to the bones. Research demonstrates that for every 100g of sugar ingested, 50mg of calcium is needed to digest it from the body's resources. Sugar intake has also been connected with an increase in osteoporosis in the hip.

BREAKFAST RECIPES

Spinach and Mushroom Omelet

Prep Time: 5mins

Cook Time: 10mins

Serving: 1

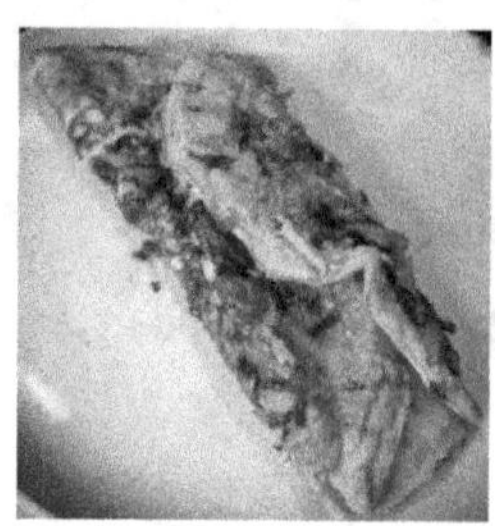

Ingredients:

2 large eggs

1 cup fresh spinach, chopped

½ cup mushrooms, sliced

2 tbsp shredded cheese (calcium-fortified if available)

1 tbsp olive oil

Salt and pepper to taste

Instructions:

- Heat olive oil in a pan over medium heat. Sauté mushrooms until tender, about 3 minutes.

- Add spinach and cook until wilted, about 2 minutes. Remove vegetables from the pan.

- In a bowl, whisk the eggs with salt and pepper. Pour into the pan, cooking over medium heat.

- Once the eggs begin to set, add the cooked vegetables and cheese on one half. Fold the omelet over and cook until the cheese is melted.

Nutritional Information (approximate):

Calories: 300

Calcium: 200mg

Vitamin D: Depending on egg fortification

Protein: 20g

Calcium-Fortified Oatmeal with Almonds and Berries

Prep Time: 5 minutes

Cook Time: 5 minutes

Servings: 1

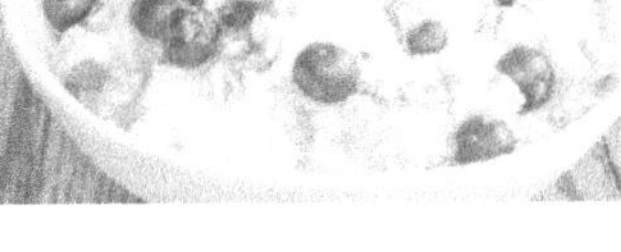

Ingredients:

½ cup rolled oats

1 cup fortified almond milk (or any fortified plant-based milk)

¼ cup blueberries

2 tbsp almonds, chopped

1 tbsp honey or maple syrup

A pinch of salt

Instructions:

- In a pot, bring the fortified almond milk to a boil. Add oats and salt, reducing heat to simmer.
- Cook until oats are soft and the mixture has thickened, about 5 minutes.
- Serve topped with blueberries, almonds, and a drizzle of honey or maple syrup.

Nutritional Information (approximate):

Calories: 350

Calcium: 300mg

Vitamin D: Depends on milk fortification

Protein: 10g

Greek Yogurt Parfait with Flaxseeds and Mixed Berries

Prep Time: 5 minutes

Cook Time: 0 minutes

Servings: 1

Ingredients:

1 cup Greek yogurt (low-fat)

½ cup mixed berries (strawberries, blueberries, raspberries)

2 tbsp ground flaxseeds

1 tbsp honey or maple syrup (optional)

Instructions:

- In a serving bowl or glass, layer Greek yogurt and mixed berries.
- Top with ground flaxseeds and a drizzle of honey or maple syrup if desired.

Nutritional Information (approximate):

Calories: 280

Calcium: 250mg

Vitamin D: Depends on yogurt fortification

Protein: 20g

Whole Grain Toast with Ricotta and Avocado

Prep Time: 5 minutes

Cook Time: 2 minutes

Servings: 1

Ingredients:

2 slices of whole-grain bread

¼ cup ricotta cheese

½ avocado, sliced

Salt and pepper to taste

Red pepper flakes (optional)

Instructions:

- Toast the whole-grain bread to your liking.
- Spread ricotta cheese evenly over the toasted slices.
- Top with avocado slices, and season with salt, pepper, and red pepper flakes if desired.

Nutritional Information (approximate):

Calories: 400

Vitamin D: 0 IU (unless using fortified bread)

Calcium: 150mg

Protein: 15g

Quinoa Breakfast Bowl with Nuts and Bananas

Prep Time: 5 minutes (if using pre-cooked quinoa)

Cook Time: 15 minutes

Servings: 1

Ingredients:

½ cup quinoa (rinsed)

1 banana, sliced

1 cup water

2 tbsp walnuts, chopped

¼ tsp cinnamon   1 tbsp honey or maple syrup

Instructions:

- In a small pot, bring water to a boil. Add quinoa and reduce to a simmer, covering until all water is absorbed, about 15 minutes.
- Fluff quinoa with a fork and transfer to a bowl.
- Top with banana slices, walnuts, and cinnamon. Drizzle with honey or maple syrup.

Nutritional Information (approximate):

Calories: 450

Calcium: 30mg

Vitamin D: 0 IU

Protein: 12g

Spicy Pumpkin Parfait

Prep Time: 10 minutes

Cook Time: 0 minutes

Servings: 1

<h2 style="text-align:center;">Ingredients:</h2>

- 1 cup Greek yogurt (low-fat, high in calcium and protein)
- ½ cup canned pumpkin puree (rich in magnesium and potassium)
- ¼ teaspoon ground cinnamon
- A pinch of ground nutmeg
- A pinch of ground ginger
- 2 tablespoons granola (preferably with nuts for added magnesium and omega-3 fatty acids)
- 1 tablespoon honey or maple syrup (optional, for sweetness)
- 2 tablespoons chopped pecans or walnuts (for healthy fats and additional magnesium)

Instructions:

- In a bowl, mix the pumpkin puree with cinnamon, nutmeg, and ginger until well combined.
- In a serving glass or jar, layer half of the Greek yogurt at the bottom.
- Add half of the pumpkin mixture over the yogurt.

- Sprinkle one tablespoon of granola and one tablespoon of chopped nuts on top of the pumpkin layer.

- Repeat the layers with the remaining yogurt, pumpkin mixture, and granola.

- Top with the remaining chopped nuts and drizzle with honey or maple syrup if desired.

- Enjoy immediately for the best texture of granola.

Nutritional Information (approximate):

- Calories: 350-400

- Calcium: 300mg

- Magnesium: 60mg

- Protein: 20g

- Vitamin D: Varies (check yogurt packaging for fortification)

Sweet Potato Pie Smoothie

Prep Time: 5mins

Cook Time: 0mins

Serving: 1

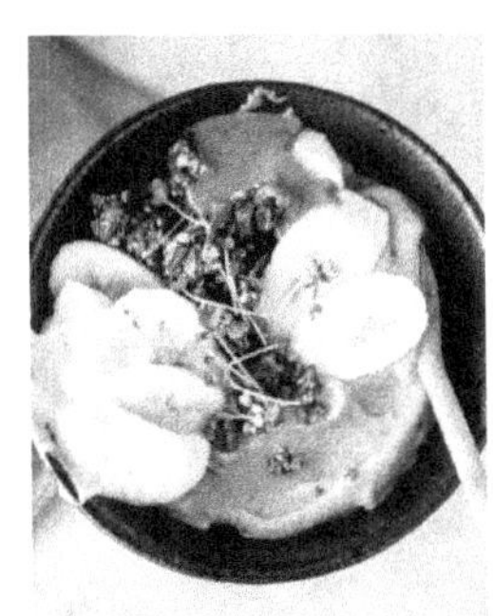

Ingredients:

- ½ cup cooked sweet potato, cooled and peeled
- 1 cup low-fat milk (dairy or fortified plant-based for calcium and vitamin D)
- ½ cup Greek yogurt (rich in calcium and protein)
- ¼ teaspoon ground cinnamon
- A pinch of ground nutmeg
- A pinch of ground ginger
- 1 tablespoon almond butter (for healthy fats and additional calcium)
- 1 tablespoon maple syrup or honey (optional, for sweetness)
- Ice cubes (optional, for texture)

Instructions:

- Place the cooked sweet potato, milk, Greek yogurt, cinnamon, nutmeg, ginger, almond butter, and sweetener (if using) into a blender.
- Add a handful of ice cubes if you prefer a colder, thicker smoothie.
- Blend on high until smooth and creamy.
- Taste and adjust sweetness if necessary.

- Pour into a glass and sprinkle a little extra cinnamon on top for garnish.

Nutritional Information (approximate):

- Calories: 350-400
- Calcium: 300-350mg
- Magnesium: 50mg
- Protein: 15-20g
- Vitamin D: Varies (check milk and yogurt packaging for fortification)

Cucumber Yogurt Salad

Prep Time: 10 minutes

Cook Time: 0 minutes

Servings: 2

Ingredients:

- 2 medium cucumbers, thinly sliced
- 1 cup Greek yogurt (low-fat, rich in calcium and protein)
- 1 clove garlic, minced (optional for extra flavor)
- 2 tablespoons fresh dill, chopped (or mint for a different flavor profile)

- 1 tablespoon lemon juice

- Salt and pepper to taste

- 1 tablespoon olive oil (for healthy fats)

- 2 tablespoons walnuts or almonds, chopped (for a crunch and a boost in magnesium and omega-3 fatty acids)

Instructions:

- In a large bowl, combine the sliced cucumbers, Greek yogurt, minced garlic, chopped dill or mint, and lemon juice. Mix until the cucumbers are well-coated with the yogurt.

- Season with salt and pepper to taste, and drizzle with olive oil. Mix gently.

- Refrigerate for at least 30 minutes before serving to allow the flavors to meld.

- Serve chilled, garnished with chopped walnuts or almonds on top for added texture and nutrients.

Nutritional Information (approximate per serving):

- Calories: 200-250

- Calcium: 150-200mg

- Magnesium: 30-40mg

- Protein: 10-15g

- Vitamin D: Varies (check yogurt packaging for fortification)

Pineapple Green Smoothie

Prep Time: 5 minutes

Cook Time: 0 minutes

Servings: 1

Ingredients:

- 1 cup fresh spinach leaves (rich in calcium, magnesium, and vitamin K)
- 1/2 cup frozen pineapple chunks (for sweetness and vitamin C)
- 1/2 banana (for creaminess and potassium)
- 1/2 cup Greek yogurt (low-fat, rich in calcium and protein)
- 1/2 cup fortified almond milk (or any fortified plant-based milk for additional calcium and vitamin D)
- 1 tablespoon chia seeds (for omega-3 fatty acids and calcium)
- A few ice cubes (optional, for a colder texture)

Instructions:

- In a blender, combine the spinach, pineapple chunks, banana, Greek yogurt, fortified almond milk, and chia seeds.

- Add ice cubes if desired for a thicker, colder smoothie.

- Blend on high until smooth and creamy. If the smoothie is too thick, add a little more almond milk until you reach your desired consistency.

- Taste and adjust sweetness if necessary, adding a bit more banana or pineapple as needed.

- Pour into a large glass and enjoy immediately for the freshest flavor and texture.

Nutritional Information (approximate):

- Calories: 300-350
- Calcium: 250-300mg
- Magnesium: 50-60mg
- Protein: 15-20g
- Vitamin D: Varies (depending on the fortification of the almond milk)

Pesto Ravioli with Spinach and Tomatoes

Prep Time: 10 minutes

Cook Time: 10 minutes

Servings: 2

Ingredients:

- 9 oz (about 250g) whole wheat or spinach ravioli (choose a variety filled with cheese for added calcium)
- 2 cups fresh spinach leaves (rich in vitamin K and calcium)
- 1 cup cherry tomatoes, halved (for vitamin C and lycopene)
- 2 tablespoons pesto sauce (homemade or store-bought, rich in healthy fats and vitamin E)
- 1 tablespoon olive oil (for healthy fats)
- Salt and pepper to taste
- Grated Parmesan cheese for garnish (additional calcium source)
- Optional: pine nuts or walnuts for garnish (for omega-3 fatty acids and magnesium)

Instructions:

- Cook the ravioli according to package instructions in a large pot of boiling salted water. Drain and set aside, reserving a little cooking water.

- While the ravioli cooks, heat olive oil in a large skillet over medium heat. Add the spinach and cherry tomatoes, sautéing until the spinach is wilted and the tomatoes are slightly softened, about 3-5 minutes.
- Add the cooked ravioli to the skillet with the spinach and tomatoes. Toss gently to combine, adding a splash of the reserved pasta water if needed to help the pesto sauce coat the ravioli evenly.
- Stir in the pesto sauce until everything is well combined and heated through. Season with salt and pepper to taste.
- Divide the ravioli among plates. Garnish with grated Parmesan cheese and optional nuts.
- Serve immediately, enjoying the blend of flavors and nutrients.

Nutritional Information (approximate per serving):

- Calories: 400-450
- Calcium: 200-250mg
- Magnesium: 50mg
- Protein: 15-20g
- Vitamin D: 0 IU (unless using fortified ingredients)

LUNCH RECIPES

Quinoa and Black Bean Salad

Prep Time: 15 minutes

Cook Time: 20 minutes

Servings: 4

Ingredients:

1 cup quinoa, rinsed

2 cups water

1 can (15 oz) black beans, drained and rinsed

1 cup cherry tomatoes, halved

1 avocado, diced

1/2 cup corn (fresh or frozen)

1/4 cup red onion, finely chopped

1/4 cup cilantro, chopped

Juice of 1 lime

2 tablespoons olive oil

Salt and pepper to taste

Instructions:

- In a medium saucepan, bring the quinoa and water to a boil. Reduce heat to low, cover, and simmer until quinoa is tender and water is absorbed, about 15 minutes. Let it cool.

- In a large bowl, combine cooled quinoa, black beans, cherry tomatoes, avocado, corn, red onion, and cilantro.
- In a small bowl, whisk together lime juice, olive oil, salt, and pepper. Pour over the salad and toss to combine.
- Serve chilled or at room temperature.

Nutritional Information (approximate per serving):

Calories: 350

Calcium: 60mg

Protein: 12g

Magnesium: 120mg

Fiber: 10g

Mediterranean Chickpea Wrap

Prep Time: 10 minutes

Cook Time: 0 minutes

Servings: 2

Ingredients:

2 whole grain wraps

1/2 cup cucumber, diced

1 cup chickpeas, rinsed and drained

1/2 cup tomatoes, diced

1/4 cup red onion, thinly sliced

1/4 cup feta cheese, crumbled

2 tablespoons hummus

1 tablespoon olive oil

1 teaspoon lemon juice

Salt and pepper to taste

Spinach leaves

Instructions:

- Lay out the wraps and spread hummus evenly on each.
- In a bowl, mix chickpeas, cucumber, tomatoes, red onion, feta cheese, olive oil, lemon juice, salt, and pepper.
- Divide the mixture between the wraps, placing it over the hummus. Add spinach leaves.
- Roll up the wraps tightly and cut in half. Serve immediately.

Nutritional Information (approximate per serving):

Calories: 400

Protein: 15g

Fiber: 8g

Calcium: 150mg

Magnesium: 80mg

Tuna and White Bean Salad

Prep Time: 10 minutes

Cook Time: 0 minutes

Servings: 2

Ingredients:

1 can (5 oz) tuna in water, drained

1 can (15 oz) white beans, drained and rinsed

1/2 red bell pepper, diced

1/4 cup red onion, finely chopped

2 tablespoons capers, rinsed

2 tablespoons olive oil

1 tablespoon lemon juice

Salt and pepper to taste

Mixed greens for serving

Instructions:

- In a bowl, combine tuna, white beans, red bell pepper, red onion, and capers.
- Drizzle with olive oil and lemon juice. Season with salt and pepper to taste. Toss to combine.
- Serve over a bed of mixed greens.

Nutritional Information (approximate per serving):

Calories: 350

Protein: 25g

Fiber: 8g

Calcium: 100mg

Magnesium: 85mg

Grilled Chicken and Vegetable Quinoa Bowl

Prep Time: 15 minutes

Cook Time: 20 minutes

Servings: 2

Ingredients:

2 boneless, skinless chicken breasts

1 cup quinoa

2 cups water

1 zucchini, sliced

1 bell pepper, sliced

1 tablespoon olive oil

2 tablespoons balsamic vinegar

Salt and pepper to taste

1/4 cup feta cheese, crumbled

Instructions:

- Grill chicken breasts seasoned with salt and pepper until cooked through. Let rest before slicing.
- Cook quinoa in water according to package instructions; set aside to cool.
- Toss zucchini and bell pepper with olive oil and grill until tender.

- In a bowl, combine quinoa, grilled vegetables, and sliced chicken. Drizzle with balsamic vinegar and add feta cheese on top.
- Serve warm or at room temperature.

Nutritional Information (approximate per serving):

Calories: 450

Calcium: 100mg

Protein: 35g

Magnesium: 150mg

Fiber: 7g

Broccoli and Almond Soup

Prep Time: 10 minutes

Cook Time: 20 minutes

Servings: 4

Ingredients:

1 tablespoon olive oil

4 cups vegetable broth

1 onion, chopped

1/2 cup almonds, toasted and chopped

2 cloves garlic, minced

4 cups broccoli florets

Salt and pepper to taste

1/2 cup light cream   (optional, for richness)

Instructions:

- In a large pot, heat olive oil over medium heat. Add onion and garlic, sautéing until softened.
- Add broccoli and vegetable broth. Bring to a boil, then reduce heat and simmer until broccoli is tender, about 15 minutes.
- Puree the soup with an immersion blender until smooth. Stir in light cream if using. Season with salt and pepper.
- Serve hot, garnished with toasted almonds.

Nutritional Information (approximate per serving):

- Calories: 200
- Protein: 6g
- Fiber: 5g
- Calcium: 80mg
- Magnesium: 75mg

Chicken and broccoli casserole

Prep Time: 20 minutes

Cook Time: 30 minutes

Servings: 4

Ingredients:

- 2 cups cooked chicken breast, shredded
- 4 cups broccoli florets, lightly steamed
- 1 cup low-fat milk (dairy or fortified plant-based for calcium and vitamin D)
- 1 cup low-fat Greek yogurt (for extra calcium and protein)
- 1/2 cup low-sodium chicken broth
- 1 teaspoon garlic powder
- 1 teaspoon onion powder
- 1/2 cup whole wheat breadcrumbs
- 1/2 cup grated Parmesan cheese (for calcium)
- 1 tablespoon olive oil
- Salt and pepper to taste

Instructions:

- Preheat the oven to 375°F (190°C). Lightly grease a 9x13 inch baking dish with olive oil.
- In a large bowl, mix together the shredded chicken and lightly steamed broccoli.
- In another bowl, whisk together the milk, Greek yogurt, chicken broth, garlic powder, and onion powder. Season with salt and pepper to taste.

- Pour the creamy mixture over the chicken and broccoli in the baking dish, stirring to ensure everything is evenly coated.
- In a small bowl, mix the breadcrumbs with grated Parmesan cheese, then sprinkle evenly over the top of the casserole.
- Drizzle the breadcrumb topping with a little olive oil to help it brown.
- Bake in the preheated oven for 25-30 minutes, or until the casserole is bubbly and the topping is golden brown.
- Let the casserole cool for a few minutes before serving.

Nutritional Information (approximate per serving):

- Calories: 350
- Protein: 30g
- Fiber: 3g
- Calcium: 250mg
- Vitamin D: Varies (depending on the milk used)

Salmon and Spinach Quiche

Prep Time: 15 minutes

Cook Time: 35 minutes

Servings: 6

Ingredients:

1 ready-to-use pie crust (whole wheat for more fiber)

4 eggs

1 cup low-fat milk (dairy or fortified plant-based)

1 cup fresh spinach, chopped

1 cup cooked salmon, flaked

½ cup shredded low-fat cheddar cheese

¼ cup diced onions

Salt and pepper to taste

Instructions:

- Preheat the oven to 375°F (190°C). Place the pie crust in a 9-inch pie dish.
- In a bowl, whisk together eggs, milk, salt, and pepper.
- Layer the spinach, salmon, cheese, and onions on the pie crust.
- Pour the egg mixture over the filling.
- Bake for 35-40 minutes, or until the quiche is set and the crust is golden brown.
- Let cool for 5 minutes before slicing and serving.

Nutritional Information (approximate per serving):

Calories: 280

Protein: 20g

Fiber: 2g

Calcium: 180mg

Vitamin D: Varies with milk and salmon

Broccoli Almond Stir-Fry

Prep Time: 10 minutes

Cook Time: 15 minutes

Servings: 4

Ingredients:

2 tablespoons olive oil

4 cups broccoli florets

1 bell pepper, sliced

1 garlic clove, minced

2 tablespoons soy sauce (low sodium)

1 tablespoon ginger, grated

½ cup almonds, toasted and sliced

1 tablespoon sesame seeds

Instructions:

- Heat olive oil in a large skillet over medium heat.

- Add garlic and ginger, sautéing for 1 minute until fragrant.
- Add broccoli and bell pepper, cooking for 5-7 minutes until tender but still crisp.
- Stir in soy sauce and cook for another 2-3 minutes.
- Toss in toasted almonds and sprinkle with sesame seeds before serving.

Nutritional Information (approximate per serving):

Calories: 220

Calcium: 75mg

Protein: 6g

Magnesium: 80mg

Fiber: 4g

Lentil and Sweet Potato Stew

Prep Time: 15 minutes

Cook Time: 30 minutes

Servings: 6

Ingredients:

1 tablespoon olive oil

1 onion, diced

2 garlic cloves, minced

1 teaspoon cumin

1 teaspoon coriander

4 cups vegetable broth

2 cups sweet potatoes, cubed

1 cup lentils (any variety, rinsed)

1 can (14 oz) diced tomatoes

Salt and pepper to taste

2 cups spinach leaves

Instructions:

- In a large pot, heat olive oil over medium heat. Add onion and garlic, cooking until softened.
- Stir in cumin and coriander, cooking for 1 minute until fragrant.
- Add broth, sweet potatoes, lentils, and tomatoes. Bring to a boil, then reduce heat and simmer for 25 minutes, or until lentils are tender.
- Stir in spinach and cook until wilted. Season with salt and pepper to taste.
- Serve hot, with crusty bread if desired.

Nutritional Information (approximate per serving):

Calories: 200

Protein: 10g

Fiber: 8g

Calcium: 50mg

Magnesium: 80mg

Baked Cod with Parmesan Crust

Prep Time: 10 minutes

Cook Time: 15 minutes

Servings: 4

Ingredients:

4 cod fillets (6 oz each)

2 tablespoons olive oil

½ cup grated Parmesan cheese

¼ cup whole wheat breadcrumbs

1 teaspoon garlic powder

1 teaspoon paprika

Salt and pepper to taste

Lemon wedges for serving

Instructions:

- Preheat oven to 400°F (200°C). Line a baking sheet with parchment paper.
- Brush cod fillets with olive oil and season with salt and pepper.

- In a bowl, mix Parmesan, breadcrumbs, garlic powder, and paprika.
- Press the Parmesan mixture onto the top of each fillet.
- Bake for 12-15 minutes, or until the crust is golden and the fish flakes easily with a fork.
- Serve immediately with lemon wedges on the side.

Nutritional Information (approximate per serving):

Calories: 250

Calcium: 150mg

Protein: 28g

Vitamin D: Varies with cod

Fiber: 1g

Roasted Vegetable and Quinoa Salad

Prep Time: 15 minutes

Cook Time: 25 minutes

Servings: 4

Ingredients:

1 cup quinoa, rinsed

2 cups water

2 cups mixed vegetables (e.g., zucchini, bell peppers, cherry tomatoes), chopped

1 tablespoon olive oil

1 teaspoon Italian seasoning

Salt and pepper to taste

2 tablespoons balsamic vinegar

¼ cup feta cheese, crumbled

¼ cup pine nuts, toasted

Instructions:

- Preheat oven to 425°F (220°C). Toss vegetables with olive oil, Italian seasoning, salt, and pepper. Spread on a baking sheet and roast for 20 minutes until tender.
- Meanwhile, cook quinoa in water according to package instructions. Fluff with a fork and let cool.
- In a large bowl, combine roasted vegetables, quinoa, balsamic vinegar, feta cheese, and pine nuts.
- Serve warm or at room temperature, adjusted with salt and pepper as needed.

Nutritional Information (approximate per serving):

- Calories: 320
- Protein: 10g
- Fiber: 5g
- Calcium: 100mg
- Magnesium: 120mg

Creamy Butternut Squash Soup

Prep Time: 15 minutes

Cook Time: 30 minutes

Servings: 4

Ingredients:

1 tablespoon olive oil

1 onion, chopped

2 cloves garlic, minced

1 medium butternut squash, peeled, seeded, and cubed

4 cups vegetable broth

1 cup light coconut milk

1 teaspoon curry powder (optional)

Salt and pepper to taste

Pumpkin seeds for garnish

Instructions:

- In a large pot, heat olive oil over medium heat. Add onion and garlic, sauté until soft.
- Add butternut squash and cook for a few minutes until slightly softened.

- Pour in vegetable broth and bring to a boil. Reduce heat, cover, and simmer until squash is tender, about 20 minutes.
- Blend the soup until smooth using an immersion blender. Stir in coconut milk and curry powder, then season with salt and pepper.
- Serve hot, garnished with pumpkin seeds.

Nutritional Information (approximate per serving):

Calories: 180

Calcium: 60mg

Protein: 3g

Vitamin C: 25mg

Fiber: 5g

Spinach and White Bean Soup

Prep Time: 10 minutes

Cook Time: 20 minutes

Servings: 4

Ingredients:

1 tablespoon olive oil

2 cloves garlic, minced

1 onion, diced

4 cups vegetable broth

1 can (15 oz) white beans, drained and rinsed

4 cups fresh spinach leaves

1 teaspoon dried oregano

Salt and pepper to taste

Grated Parmesan cheese for garnish

Instructions:

- Heat olive oil in a large pot over medium heat. Add onion and garlic, sauté until translucent.
- Add vegetable broth, beans, and oregano. Season with salt and pepper. Bring to a boil, then simmer for 10 minutes.
- Stir in spinach and cook until wilted, about 2 minutes.
- Serve hot, topped with grated Parmesan cheese.

Nutritional Information (approximate per serving):

Calories: 150

Protein: 8g

Fiber: 6g

Calcium: 100mg

Iron: 3mg

Tomato Basil Soup

Prep Time: 5 minutes

Cook Time: 25 minutes

Servings: 4

Ingredients:

1 tablespoon olive oil

1 onion, chopped

2 cloves garlic, minced

1 can (28 oz) crushed tomatoes

2 cups vegetable broth

1/2 cup fresh basil, chopped

1/2 cup heavy cream or coconut milk

Salt and pepper to taste

Instructions:

- In a pot, heat olive oil over medium. Sauté onion and garlic until soft.
- Add crushed tomatoes and vegetable broth. Bring to a simmer and cook for 20 minutes.
- Stir in basil and cream or coconut milk. Heat through.
- Blend until smooth. Season with salt and pepper.
- Serve garnished with more basil.

Nutritional Information (approximate per serving):

Calories: 200

Protein: 4g

Fiber: 4g

Calcium: 70mg

Vitamin A: 25% DV

Carrot Ginger Soup

Prep Time: 10 minutes

Cook Time: 30 minutes

Servings: 4

Ingredients:

2 tablespoons olive oil

1 onion, chopped

2 tablespoons fresh ginger, minced

6 carrots, peeled and chopped

4 cups vegetable broth

Salt and pepper to taste

Coconut milk for drizzling

Instructions:

Heat olive oil in a large pot. Add onion and ginger, sauté until softened.

Add carrots and vegetable broth. Bring to a boil, then simmer until carrots are tender.

Blend the soup until smooth. Season with salt and pepper.

Serve hot, drizzled with coconut milk.

Nutritional Information (approximate per serving):

Calories: 150

Calcium: 50mg

Protein: 2g

Vitamin A: 210% DV

Fiber: 4g

Lentil and Kale Soup

Prep Time: 10 minutes

Cook Time: 40 minutes

Servings: 6

Ingredients:

1 tablespoon olive oil

1 cup lentils, rinsed

1 onion, diced

6 cups vegetable broth

2 cloves garlic, minced

2 cups kale, chopped

1 carrot, diced

1 teaspoon cumin

1 stalk celery, diced

Salt and pepper to taste

Instructions:

- In a large pot, heat olive oil. Add onion, garlic, carrot, and celery. Cook until softened.
- Add lentils, vegetable broth, and cumin. Season with salt and pepper.
- Bring to a boil, then reduce heat and simmer until lentils are tender, about 30 minutes.
- Stir in kale and cook until wilted, about 10 minutes.
- Serve hot, adjusting seasoning as needed.

Nutritional Information (approximate per serving):

Calories: 200

Calcium: 80mg

Protein: 12g

Iron: 3.5mg

Fiber: 8g

Roasted Red Pepper and Tomato Soup

Prep Time: 10 minutes

Cook Time: 30 minutes

Servings: 4

Ingredients:

2 tablespoons olive oil

1 onion, chopped

2 cloves garlic, minced

4 roasted red peppers, chopped (jarred or homemade)

1 can (28 oz) diced tomatoes, undrained

2 cups vegetable broth

1 teaspoon smoked paprika

Salt and pepper to taste

Fresh basil for garnish

Optional: dollop of Greek yogurt for serving

Instructions:

- In a large pot, heat olive oil over medium heat. Add onion and garlic, sauté until translucent.
- Stir in roasted red peppers, diced tomatoes with their juice, vegetable broth, and smoked paprika. Season with salt and pepper.
- Bring to a boil, then reduce heat and simmer for 20 minutes.
- Puree the soup with an immersion blender until smooth.
- Serve hot, garnished with fresh basil and an optional dollop of Greek yogurt.

Nutritional Information (approximate per serving):

Calories: 150

Protein: 3g

Fiber: 4g

Vitamin C: 120mg

Calcium: 50mg

Creamy Mushroom and Wild Rice Soup

Prep Time: 15 minutes

Cook Time: 45 minutes

Servings: 4

Ingredients:

1 tablespoon olive oil

1 onion, diced

2 cloves garlic, minced

1 pound mushrooms, sliced
(mix of button and wild
mushrooms)

1 cup wild rice, rinsed

4 cups vegetable broth

1 cup light cream or
coconut milk

2 teaspoons thyme

Salt and pepper to taste

Chopped parsley for garnish

Instructions:

- In a large pot, heat olive oil over medium heat. Add onion, garlic, and mushrooms, cooking until mushrooms are browned.
- Stir in wild rice, vegetable broth, and thyme. Season with salt and pepper.
- Bring to a boil, then reduce heat, cover, and simmer until rice is tender, about 45 minutes.
- Stir in light cream or coconut milk, heating through.
- Serve garnished with chopped parsley.

Nutritional Information (approximate per serving):

Calories: 250

Calcium: 60mg

Protein: 8g

Vitamin D: 0 IU (unless using fortified ingredients)

Fiber: 3g

Sweet Potato and Lentil Soup

Prep Time: 15 minutes

Cook Time: 30 minutes

Servings: 4

Ingredients:

1 tablespoon olive oil

1 onion, chopped

2 cloves garlic, minced

4 cups vegetable broth

2 sweet potatoes, peeled and cubed

1 teaspoon cumin

Salt and pepper to taste

1 cup red lentils, rinsed

Fresh cilantro for garnish

Instructions:

- In a large pot, heat olive oil over medium heat. Add onion and garlic, sauté until soft.
- Add sweet potatoes, lentils, vegetable broth, and cumin. Season with salt and pepper.
- Bring to a boil, then reduce heat and simmer until sweet potatoes and lentils are tender, about 25 minutes.
- Puree part of the soup for a creamier texture, if desired.
- Serve garnished with fresh cilantro.

Nutritional Information (approximate per serving):

Calories: 260

Calcium: 40mg

Protein: 10g

Vitamin A: 180% DV

Fiber: 8g

Zucchini Basil Soup

Prep Time: 10 minutes

Cook Time: 20 minutes

Servings: 4

Ingredients:

2 tablespoons olive oil

2 cloves garlic, minced

4 zucchinis, chopped

4 cups vegetable broth

½ cup fresh basil, plus more for garnish

Salt and pepper to taste

Optional: shredded Parmesan cheese for serving

Instructions:

- In a large pot, heat olive oil over medium heat. Add garlic and zucchini, sauté until softened.
- Add vegetable broth and bring to a boil. Reduce heat and simmer for 10 minutes.
- Stir in fresh basil, and use an immersion blender to puree the soup until smooth.
- Season with salt and pepper to taste.
- Serve hot, garnished with more basil and optional Parmesan cheese.

Nutritional Information (approximate per serving):

Calories: 100

Protein: 2g

Fiber: 2g

Vitamin C: 35% DV

Calcium: 30mg

Cauliflower and Potato Soup

Prep Time: 10 minutes

Cook Time: 25 minutes

Servings: 4

Ingredients:

1 tablespoon olive oil

1 onion, chopped

2 cloves garlic, minced

1 head cauliflower, chopped

2 potatoes, peeled and cubed

4 cups vegetable broth

1 teaspoon thyme

Salt and pepper to taste

Optional: light cream for a creamier texture

Instructions:

- In a large pot, heat olive oil over medium heat. Add onion and garlic, cooking until translucent.

- Add cauliflower, potatoes, vegetable broth, and thyme. Season with salt and pepper.

- Bring to a boil, then reduce heat and simmer until vegetables are tender, about 20 minutes.

- Puree the soup with an immersion blender until smooth. Stir in light cream if using, and adjust seasoning.

- Serve hot, with a drizzle of olive oil or a sprinkle of thyme.

Nutritional Information (approximate per serving):

- Calories: 150
- Protein: 4g
- Fiber: 5g
- Calcium: 50mg
- Vitamin C: 80% DV

Kale and Quinoa Super Salad

Prep Time: 15 minutes

Cook Time: 20 minutes (for quinoa)

Servings: 4

Ingredients:

1 cup quinoa, rinsed

2 cups water

4 cups kale, stems removed and leaves chopped

1 avocado, diced

1/2 cup dried cranberries

1/2 cup slivered almonds, toasted

2 tablespoons olive oil

Juice of 1 lemon

Salt and pepper to taste

Optional: crumbled goat cheese for extra protein and calcium

Instructions:

- Cook quinoa in water according to package instructions. Let cool.

- In a large bowl, combine cooled quinoa, kale, avocado, dried cranberries, and almonds.
- Whisk together olive oil and lemon juice, then pour over the salad. Toss to coat evenly.
- Season with salt and pepper to taste. Garnish with goat cheese if using.
- Serve chilled or at room temperature.

Nutritional Information (approximate per serving):

Calories: 350

Calcium: 150mg

Protein: 10g

Magnesium: 100mg

Fiber: 7g

Mediterranean Chickpea Salad

Prep Time: 15 minutes

Cook Time: 0 minutes

Servings: 4

Ingredients:

2 cans (15 oz each) chickpeas, drained and rinsed

1 cucumber, diced

1 bell pepper, diced

1/2 red onion, thinly sliced

1/2 cup Kalamata olives,
pitted and halved

1 cup cherry tomatoes,
halved

1/2 cup feta cheese,
crumbled

1/4 cup olive oil

Juice of 1 lemon

2 teaspoons dried oregano

Salt and pepper to taste

Instructions:

- In a large bowl, combine chickpeas, cucumber, bell pepper, red onion, olives, and cherry tomatoes.
- Add feta cheese to the bowl.
- In a small bowl, whisk together olive oil, lemon juice, oregano, salt, and pepper. Pour over salad and toss to combine.
- Serve immediately or chill in the refrigerator for an hour to enhance flavors.

Nutritional Information (approximate per serving):

Calories: 400

Protein: 15g

Fiber: 10g

Calcium: 200mg

Magnesium: 80mg

Beet and Goat Cheese Arugula Salad

Prep Time: 10 minutes

Cook Time: 0 minutes (assuming pre-cooked beets)

Servings: 4

Ingredients:

4 cups arugula

1 cup cooked beets, sliced

1/2 cup goat cheese, crumbled

1/4 cup walnuts, toasted and chopped

2 tablespoons balsamic vinegar

2 tablespoons olive oil

Salt and pepper to taste

Optional: drizzle of honey

Instructions:

- In a large salad bowl, arrange arugula as the base.
- Top with sliced beets, crumbled goat cheese, and toasted walnuts.
- In a small bowl, whisk together balsamic vinegar and olive oil. Season with salt and pepper.
- Drizzle the dressing over the salad just before serving. Add a drizzle of honey for extra sweetness if desired.

Nutritional Information (approximate per serving):

Calories: 250

Protein: 8g

Fiber: 3g

Calcium: 100mg

Magnesium: 50mg

Asian Sesame Chicken Salad

Prep Time: 20 minutes

Cook Time: 15 minutes (for chicken)

Servings: 4

Ingredients:

2 boneless, skinless chicken breasts

4 cups mixed salad greens

1 cup red cabbage, shredded

1 carrot, julienned

1/2 cup cucumbers, thinly sliced

1/4 cup cilantro, chopped

1/4 cup toasted almonds, sliced

2 tablespoons sesame seeds

For the dressing:

1/4 cup soy sauce (low sodium)

2 tablespoons sesame oil

2 tablespoons rice vinegar

1 tablespoon honey   1 teaspoon ginger, grated

1 garlic clove, minced

Instructions:

- Grill or pan-fry chicken breasts seasoned with salt and pepper until cooked through. Let cool and then slice thinly.
- In a large salad bowl, combine salad greens, red cabbage, carrot, cucumbers, and cilantro.
- Top with sliced chicken, toasted almonds, and sesame seeds.
- In a small bowl, whisk together all dressing ingredients until well combined.
- Drizzle dressing over the salad just before serving and toss to combine.

Nutritional Information (approximate per serving):

Calories: 300   Calcium: 80mg

Protein: 25g   Magnesium: 70mg

Fiber: 4g

Strawberry Spinach Salad with Poppy Seed Dressing

Prep Time: 15 minutes

Cook Time: 0 minutes

Servings: 4

Ingredients:

4 cups spinach leaves

1 cup strawberries, sliced

1/2 cup walnuts, toasted and chopped

1/2 cup goat cheese, crumbled

For the dressing:

1/4 cup olive oil

2 tablespoons apple cider vinegar

1 tablespoon honey

1 teaspoon poppy seeds

Salt and pepper to taste

Instructions:

- In a large salad bowl, combine spinach, sliced strawberries, toasted walnuts, and crumbled goat cheese.
- In a small bowl, whisk together olive oil, apple cider vinegar, honey, poppy seeds, salt, and pepper to create the dressing.

- Drizzle the dressing over the salad just before serving and gently toss to combine.

Nutritional Information (approximate per serving):

- Calories: 250
- Protein: 8g
- Fiber: 3g
- Calcium: 100mg
- Magnesium: 40mg

Avocado and Black Bean Salad

Prep Time: 15 minutes

Cook Time: 0 minutes

Servings: 4

Ingredients:

2 ripe avocados, diced

1 can (15 oz) black beans, rinsed and drained

1 cup corn kernels (fresh, canned, or thawed from frozen)

1 red bell pepper, diced

1/4 cup red onion, finely chopped

1/4 cup cilantro, chopped

Juice of 2 limes

2 tablespoons olive oil

1 teaspoon cumin (optional)

Salt and pepper to taste

Instructions:

- In a large bowl, combine the diced avocados, black beans, corn, red bell pepper, red onion, and cilantro.
- In a small bowl, whisk together lime juice, olive oil, salt, pepper, and cumin if using, to make the dressing.
- Pour the dressing over the salad ingredients and gently toss to combine without breaking the avocado pieces.
- Serve immediately or chill in the refrigerator for 30 minutes before serving to blend the flavors.

Nutritional Information (approximate per serving):

- Calories: 300
- Protein: 8g
- Fiber: 10g
- Calcium: 50mg
- Magnesium: 70mg

Pear and Gorgonzola Salad with Walnuts

Prep Time: 10 minutes

Cook Time: 0 minutes

Servings: 4

Ingredients:

4 cups mixed greens (e.g., arugula, spinach, and romaine)

2 ripe pears, sliced

1/2 cup Gorgonzola cheese, crumbled

1/2 cup walnuts, toasted and chopped

For the dressing:

1/4 cup balsamic vinegar

1/2 cup olive oil

1 tablespoon honey

Salt and pepper to taste

Instructions:

- Arrange mixed greens in a large salad bowl.
- Top with sliced pears, Gorgonzola cheese, and toasted walnuts.
- In a small bowl, whisk together balsamic vinegar, olive oil, honey, salt, and pepper to create the dressing.
- Drizzle the dressing over the salad just before serving and toss gently to combine.

Nutritional Information (approximate per serving):

Calories: 350

Protein: 6g

Fiber: 4g

Calcium: 100mg

Magnesium: 30mg

Grilled Vegetable and Farro Salad

Prep Time: 20 minutes

Cook Time: 30 minutes

Servings: 4

Ingredients:

1 cup farro, rinsed

2 zucchinis, sliced lengthwise

1 eggplant, sliced into rounds

1 red bell pepper, sliced into strips

1/4 cup olive oil, divided

2 tablespoons balsamic vinegar

1/2 cup cherry tomatoes, halved

1/4 cup basil leaves, chopped

Salt and pepper to taste

Optional: crumbled feta or goat cheese for added flavor

Instructions:

- Cook farro in boiling water according to package instructions until tender. Drain and let cool.
- Preheat grill to medium-high heat. Toss zucchinis, eggplant, and red bell pepper with half the olive oil. Grill until charred and tender, turning occasionally.
- In a large bowl, combine grilled vegetables, cooked farro, cherry tomatoes, and basil.
- Whisk together remaining olive oil, balsamic vinegar, salt, and pepper to create the dressing.
- Pour the dressing over the salad and toss to combine. Serve at room temperature or chilled, topped with crumbled cheese if desired.

Nutritional Information (approximate per serving):

Calories: 400

Calcium: 60mg

Protein: 8g

Magnesium: 80mg

Fiber: 8g

Crunchy Cabbage and Carrot Slaw

Prep Time: 15 minutes

Cook Time: 0 minutes

Servings: 4

Ingredients:

2 cups red cabbage, thinly sliced	1/4 cup olive oil
2 cups green cabbage, thinly sliced	2 tablespoons honey
1 large carrot, julienned	1 tablespoon Dijon mustard
1/2 cup apple cider vinegar	Salt and pepper to taste
	1/4 cup sunflower seeds

Instructions:

- In a large bowl, combine red cabbage, green cabbage, and carrot.
- In a small bowl, whisk together apple cider vinegar, olive oil, honey, Dijon mustard, salt, and pepper to create the dressing.
- Pour the dressing over the cabbage mixture and toss to coat evenly.
- Let the slaw sit for at least 30 minutes in the refrigerator to marinate and soften.
- Just before serving, sprinkle with sunflower seeds for added crunch.

Nutritional Information (approximate per serving):

Calories: 200

Protein: 2g

Fiber: 3g

Calcium: 40mg

Magnesium: 30mg

Mediterranean Orzo Salad

Prep Time: 15 minutes

Cook Time: 10 minutes

Servings: 4

Ingredients:

1 cup orzo pasta

1/2 cup sun-dried tomatoes, chopped

1/2 cup Kalamata olives, pitted and sliced

1/4 cup red onion, finely chopped

1 cucumber, diced

1/2 cup feta cheese, crumbled

For the dressing:

1/4 cup olive oil

Juice of 1 lemon

1 teaspoon dried oregano

Salt and pepper to taste

Instructions:

- Cook orzo according to package instructions until al dente. Drain and rinse under cold water to cool.

- In a large bowl, combine cooled orzo with sun-dried tomatoes, olives, red onion, cucumber, and feta cheese.

- In a small bowl, whisk together olive oil, lemon juice, oregano, salt, and pepper to create the dressing.

- Pour the dressing over the orzo mixture and toss to combine.

- Chill in the refrigerator for at least 1 hour before serving to allow flavors to meld.

Nutritional Information (approximate per serving):

- Calories: 350
- Protein: 8g
- Fiber: 3g
- Calcium: 100mg
- Magnesium: 50mg

HEALTHY SNACKS FOR BONE DENSITY

Greek Yogurt and Berry Parfait

Prep Time: 5 minutes

Cook Time: 0 minutes

Servings: 1

Ingredients:

- 1 cup Greek yogurt (low-fat for calcium and protein)
- 1/2 cup mixed berries (strawberries, blueberries, raspberries for antioxidants and vitamins)
- 2 tablespoons granola (for crunch and fiber)
- 1 tablespoon honey or maple syrup (optional for sweetness)

Instructions:

- In a serving glass or bowl, layer half of the Greek yogurt at the bottom.
- Add a layer of mixed berries, then sprinkle a tablespoon of granola.
- Repeat the layers with the remaining yogurt, berries, and granola.

- Drizzle with honey or maple syrup if desired.
- Serve immediately for a fresh and nutritious snack.

Nutritional Information (approximate per serving):

Calories: 250

Fiber: 3g

Protein: 20g

Calcium: 250mg

Almond and Date Energy Balls

Prep Time: 15 minutes

Cook Time: 0 minutes (chill time 1 hour)

Servings: 12 balls

Ingredients:

1 cup almonds (for healthy fats and magnesium)

1/4 cup unsweetened cocoa powder

1 cup dates, pitted (natural sweetness and fiber)

1 tablespoon chia seeds (for omega-3s and fiber)

2 tablespoons coconut oil

Instructions:

- In a food processor, blend almonds until finely ground.

- Add dates, cocoa powder, chia seeds, and coconut oil. Process until the mixture sticks together.
- Roll the mixture into small balls, about 1 inch in diameter.
- Place the balls on a baking sheet lined with parchment paper and refrigerate for at least 1 hour to set.
- Store in an airtight container in the refrigerator.

Nutritional Information (approximate per serving):

Calories: 150

Fiber: 3g

Protein: 4g

Calcium: 40mg

Avocado Toast with Pumpkin Seeds

Prep Time: 5 minutes

Cook Time: 2 minutes

Servings: 1

Ingredients:

- 1 slice whole-grain bread (toasted for fiber and nutrients)
- 1/2 ripe avocado (for healthy fats and vitamin E)
- Salt and pepper to taste
- 1 tablespoon pumpkin seeds (for magnesium and omega-3s)

Instructions:

- Mash the avocado in a small bowl and season with salt and pepper.
- Spread the mashed avocado evenly over the toasted bread.
- Sprinkle pumpkin seeds on top.
- Serve immediately for a crunchy, creamy snack.

Nutritional Information (approximate per serving):

Calories: 250

Fiber: 7g

Protein: 6g

Calcium: 30mg

Cottage Cheese and Fruit Bowl

Prep Time: 5 minutes

Cook Time: 0 minutes

Servings: 1

Ingredients:

- 1 cup low-fat cottage cheese (for calcium and protein)
- 1/2 cup sliced peaches or any preferred fruit (for vitamins and fiber)
- 1 tablespoon flaxseeds (for omega-3s and fiber)

Instructions:

- Place the cottage cheese in a serving bowl.
- Top with sliced peaches or your choice of fruit.
- Sprinkle flaxseeds over the top.
- Mix gently before eating, if desired.

Nutritional Information (approximate per serving):

Calories: 200

Fiber: 4g

Protein: 28g

Calcium: 150mg

Veggie Sticks with Hummus

Prep Time: 10 minutes

Cook Time: 0 minutes

Servings: 2

Ingredients:

1/2 cup hummus (for protein and fiber)

1 carrot, cut into sticks

1 cucumber, cut into sticks

1 bell pepper, cut into sticks

1/4 cup broccoli florets

Instructions:

- Arrange the carrot, cucumber, bell pepper sticks, and broccoli florets on a plate or in a serving container.
- Serve with hummus for dipping.
- Enjoy a refreshing and filling snack that's perfect for any time of the day.

Nutritional Information (approximate per serving):

Calories: 150

Protein: 6g

Fiber: 5g

Calcium: 50mg

Baked Sweet Potato Chips

Prep Time: 10 minutes

Cook Time: 20 minutes

Servings: 4

Ingredients:

2 large sweet potatoes, thinly sliced

1 tablespoon olive oil

Salt and pepper to taste

Optional: paprika or cinnamon for extra flavor

Instructions:

- Preheat oven to 400°F (200°C). Line a baking sheet with parchment paper.
- Toss the sweet potato slices with olive oil, salt, pepper, and any additional spices until evenly coated.
- Arrange the slices in a single layer on the baking sheet.
- Bake for 10 minutes, flip the chips, and continue baking for another 10 minutes or until crispy.
- Let cool before serving to achieve maximum crispiness.

Nutritional Information (approximate per serving):

Calories: 120

Fiber: 3g

Protein: 2g

Calcium: 40mg

Roasted Chickpeas

Prep Time: 5 minutes

Cook Time: 40 minutes

Servings: 4

Ingredients:

1 can (15 oz) chickpeas, drained, rinsed, and dried

1 tablespoon olive oil

1/2 teaspoon salt

Optional: spices such as cumin, smoked paprika, or garlic powder

Instructions:

- Preheat oven to 375°F (190°C).
- Toss chickpeas with olive oil, salt, and any desired spices until evenly coated.
- Spread the chickpeas in a single layer on a baking sheet.
- Roast for 30-40 minutes, stirring occasionally, until crispy and golden.
- Cool before serving to enhance crunchiness.

Nutritional Information (approximate per serving):

Calories: 150

Protein: 6g

Fiber: 5g

Calcium: 50mg

Peanut Butter Banana Bites

Prep Time: 15 minutes (plus freezing time)

Cook Time: 0 minutes

Servings: 4

Ingredients:

2 bananas, sliced into rounds

1/4 cup natural peanut butter

1/2 cup dark chocolate chips, melted

Optional toppings: crushed nuts, coconut flakes

Instructions:

- Sandwich a small amount of peanut butter between two banana slices.
- Dip half of the banana bites into melted dark chocolate, then sprinkle with optional toppings.
- Place on a baking sheet lined with parchment paper and freeze until solid, about 2 hours.
- Store in an airtight container in the freezer.

Nutritional Information (approximate per serving):

- Calories: 200
- Protein: 4g
- Fiber: 3g
- Calcium: 20mg

Cucumber Roll-Ups

Prep Time: 15 minutes

Cook Time: 0 minutes

Servings: 4

Ingredients:

2 large cucumbers, thinly sliced lengthwise

1 cup hummus

1/2 cup shredded carrots

1/2 bell pepper, thinly sliced

1/4 cup feta cheese, crumbled

1 tablespoon lemon juice

Salt and pepper to taste

Instructions:

- Spread a thin layer of hummus over each cucumber slice.
- Top with shredded carrots, bell pepper slices, and a sprinkle of feta cheese.
- Drizzle with lemon juice and season with salt and pepper.
- Carefully roll up the cucumber slices and secure with a toothpick.

- Serve chilled as a fresh, crunchy snack.

Nutritional Information (approximate per serving):

Calories: 150

Fiber: 4g

Protein: 6g

Calcium: 60mg

Greek Yogurt with Honey and Walnuts

Prep Time: 5 minutes

Cook Time: 0 minutes

Servings: 1

Ingredients:

- 1 cup Greek yogurt (low-fat for calcium and protein)
- 2 tablespoons walnuts, chopped (for omega-3 fatty acids and antioxidants)
- 1 tablespoon honey (for natural sweetness)
- **Optional: sprinkle of cinnamon**

Instructions:

- Spoon Greek yogurt into a serving bowl.
- Top with chopped walnuts and a drizzle of honey.

- Add a sprinkle of cinnamon if desired.

- Mix gently before eating.

Nutritional Information (approximate per serving):

- Calories: 250

- Protein: 20g

- Fiber: 2g

- Calcium: 250mg

HEALTHY DESSERT FOR BONE DENSITY

Avocado Chocolate Mousse

Prep Time: 10 minutes

Cook Time: 0 minutes

Chill Time: 1 hour

Servings: 4

Ingredients:

2 ripe avocados, peeled and
pitted

1/4 cup cocoa powder

1/4 cup honey or maple
syrup

1/2 teaspoon vanilla extract

Pinch of salt

Optional toppings: berries,
coconut flakes, or chopped
nuts

Instructions:

- In a blender or food processor, combine avocados, cocoa powder, honey or maple syrup, vanilla extract, and salt. Blend until smooth and creamy.
- Divide the mousse into serving dishes and refrigerate for at least 1 hour to set.
- Garnish with optional toppings before serving.

Nutritional Information (approximate per serving):

Calories: 220

Protein: 3g

Fiber: 7g

Calcium: 20mg

Baked Apple Slices with Cinnamon

Prep Time: 10 minutes

Cook Time: 20 minutes

Servings: 4

Ingredients:

- 4 apples, cored and sliced
- 2 tablespoons honey or maple syrup
- 1/2 teaspoon ground cinnamon
- Juice of 1/2 lemon

Instructions:

- Preheat the oven to 375°F (190°C). Line a baking sheet with parchment paper.
- In a large bowl, toss apple slices with honey or maple syrup, cinnamon, and lemon juice until well coated.
- Arrange apple slices in a single layer on the prepared baking sheet.
- Bake for 20 minutes or until apples are tender and slightly caramelized.
- Serve warm, perhaps with a dollop of Greek yogurt for extra protein.

Nutritional Information (approximate per serving):

- Calories: 120
- Protein: 0.5g
- Fiber: 4g

- Calcium: 10mg

No-Bake Peanut Butter Oat Bars

Prep Time: 15 minutes

Chill Time: 1 hour

Servings: 12 bars

Ingredients:

1 cup natural peanut butter

1/2 cup honey or maple syrup

2 cups rolled oats

1/2 cup mini dark chocolate chips

Pinch of salt

Instructions:

- In a saucepan over medium heat, melt together peanut butter and honey or maple syrup.
- Remove from heat and stir in rolled oats, chocolate chips, and a pinch of salt until well combined.
- Press the mixture into a lined 8x8 inch baking pan.
- Refrigerate for at least 1 hour until set.
- Cut into bars and serve.

Nutritional Information (approximate per serving):

Calories: 250

Fiber: 3g

Protein: 7g

Calcium: 20mg

Mixed Berry Yogurt Parfait

Prep Time: 10 minutes

Cook Time: 0 minutes

Servings: 4

Ingredients:

2 cups Greek yogurt (low-fat for calcium and protein)

2 cups mixed berries (strawberries, blueberries, raspberries)

1/4 cup granola

Honey or maple syrup to taste

Instructions:

- In serving glasses, layer Greek yogurt, mixed berries, and granola. Repeat layers until glasses are filled.
- Drizzle with honey or maple syrup to taste.
- Serve immediately or chill in the refrigerator until ready to serve.

Nutritional Information (approximate per serving):

Calories: 200	Fiber: 3g
Protein: 15g	Calcium: 150mg

Coconut Rice Pudding

Prep Time: 5 minutes

Cook Time: 45 minutes

Servings: 6

Ingredients:

1 cup Arborio rice

1 can (14 oz) coconut milk

2 cups milk (dairy or fortified plant-based)

1/3 cup sugar

1/2 teaspoon vanilla extract

Pinch of salt

Optional: mango slices or toasted coconut flakes for topping

Instructions:

- In a large saucepan, combine Arborio rice, coconut milk, milk, sugar, vanilla extract, and a pinch of salt.
- Bring to a boil, then reduce heat to low and simmer, stirring frequently, until the rice is tender and the mixture is creamy, about 45 minutes.

- Remove from heat and let cool slightly. The pudding will thicken as it cools.
- Serve warm or chilled, topped with mango slices or toasted coconut flakes if desired.

Nutritional Information (approximate per serving):

Calories: 300

Fiber: 1g

Protein: 5g

Calcium: 100mg

Lemon Chia Seed Pudding

Prep Time: 5 minutes (plus at least 4 hours chilling)

Cook Time: 0 minutes

Servings: 4

Ingredients:

2 cups almond milk (or any fortified plant-based milk)

1/2 cup chia seeds

1/4 cup maple syrup or honey

Zest of 1 lemon

Juice of 1 lemon

Optional toppings: fresh berries, sliced almonds

Instructions:

- In a mixing bowl, whisk together almond milk, chia seeds, maple syrup or honey, lemon zest, and lemon juice until well combined.
- Divide the mixture evenly among serving glasses or bowls.
- Refrigerate for at least 4 hours, or overnight, until the pudding has thickened.
- Before serving, stir the pudding to ensure a uniform texture and garnish with fresh berries and sliced almonds if desired.

Nutritional Information (approximate per serving):

Calories: 180

Fiber: 10g

Protein: 5g

Calcium: 300mg (if using fortified almond milk)

Frozen Yogurt Bark with Mixed Berries

Prep Time: 5 minutes (plus freezing time)

Cook Time: 0 minutes

Servings: 8

Ingredients:

2 cups Greek yogurt (low-fat for calcium and protein)

2 tablespoons honey or maple syrup

1/2 cup mixed berries (such as strawberries, blueberries, and raspberries)

2 tablespoons dark chocolate chips

1 tablespoon shredded coconut

Instructions:

- Line a baking sheet with parchment paper.
- In a bowl, mix the Greek yogurt with honey or maple syrup.
- Spread the yogurt mixture evenly onto the prepared baking sheet.
- Sprinkle with mixed berries, dark chocolate chips, and shredded coconut.
- Freeze for at least 4 hours or until firm.
- Break or cut into pieces and serve immediately.

Nutritional Information (approximate per serving):

Calories: 100

Protein: 6g

Fiber: 1g

Calcium: 150mg

Pear and Ricotta Cheese Plate

Prep Time: 5 minutes

Cook Time: 0 minutes

Servings: 4

Ingredients:

2 ripe pears, sliced

1 cup ricotta cheese (part-skim for calcium and protein)

2 tablespoons honey

1/4 cup walnuts, chopped

Optional: cinnamon or nutmeg for sprinkling

Instructions:

- Arrange the sliced pears on a serving plate.
- Dollop ricotta cheese alongside the pear slices.
- Drizzle honey over the pears and ricotta.
- Sprinkle with chopped walnuts and a dash of cinnamon or nutmeg if desired.
- Serve immediately as a fresh and satisfying dessert or snack.

Nutritional Information (approximate per serving):

Calories: 200

Protein: 8g

Fiber: 3g   Calcium: 200mg

. Chocolate-Dipped Strawberry Skewers

Prep Time: 15 minutes (plus chilling)

Cook Time: 2 minutes

Servings: 6

Ingredients:

- 1 pound strawberries, washed and dried
- 8 ounces dark chocolate, chopped
- Optional toppings: crushed nuts, coconut flakes, or sea salt

Instructions:

- Thread strawberries onto skewers.
- Melt dark chocolate in a double boiler or in the microwave, stirring until smooth.
- Dip each strawberry skewer into the melted chocolate, coating as desired.
- Lay the dipped skewers on a baking sheet lined with parchment paper.
- Sprinkle with optional toppings if using.
- Refrigerate until the chocolate is set, about 30 minutes.

- Serve chilled.

Nutritional Information (approximate per serving):

Calories: 200

Fiber: 3g

Protein: 2g

Calcium: 20mg

Baked Cinnamon Apple Chips

Prep Time: 10 minutes

Cook Time: 2-3 hours

Servings: 4

Ingredients:

- 2 large apples, thinly sliced
- 1 teaspoon ground cinnamon
- Optional: sugar or sugar substitute for sprinkling

Instructions:

- Preheat oven to 200°F (93°C). Line two baking sheets with parchment paper.
- Arrange apple slices in a single layer on the baking sheets.

- Sprinkle apple slices with cinnamon, and if desired, a light sprinkle of sugar.
- Bake for 2-3 hours, flipping the slices halfway through, until the apple slices are dried out and crisp.
- Let cool completely before serving. Store in an airtight container.

Nutritional Information (approximate per serving):

- Calories: 50
- Protein: 0g
- Fiber: 4g
- Calcium: 10mg

SMOOTHIE RECIPES

Green Power Smoothie

Prep Time: 5 minutes

Cook Time: 0 minutes

Servings: 2

Ingredients:

2 cups fresh spinach

1 ripe banana, sliced

1/2 avocado, peeled and pitted

1 cup unsweetened almond milk (or any plant-based milk)

1 tablespoon chia seeds

1 tablespoon honey (optional)

Ice cubes (optional)

Instructions:

- Place spinach, banana, avocado, almond milk, chia seeds, and honey (if using) in a blender.
- Blend on high until smooth. Add ice cubes to achieve a thicker consistency, if desired.

- Serve immediately, garnished with a sprinkle of chia seeds on top for extra crunch.

Nutritional Information (approximate per serving):

Calories: 200

Fiber: 7g

Protein: 4g

Calcium: 150mg (if using fortified almond milk)

Berry Antioxidant Smoothie

Prep Time: 5 minutes

Cook Time: 0 minutes

Servings: 2

Ingredients:

1 cup frozen mixed berries (strawberries, blueberries, raspberries)

1 banana, sliced

1 cup Greek yogurt (low-fat for calcium and protein)

1/2 cup orange juice

1 tablespoon flaxseed meal

Ice cubes (optional)

Instructions:

- Combine mixed berries, banana, Greek yogurt, orange juice, and flaxseed meal in a blender.
- Blend on high until creamy and smooth. Add ice cubes for a colder, thicker smoothie, if desired.
- Pour into glasses and serve immediately.

Nutritional Information (approximate per serving):

Calories: 220

Fiber: 4g

Protein: 10g

Calcium: 200mg

Tropical Mango Pineapple Smoothie

Prep Time: 5 minutes

Cook Time: 0 minutes

Servings: 2

Ingredients:

1 cup frozen mango chunks

1 banana, sliced

1 cup frozen pineapple chunks

1 cup coconut water

1/2 cup Greek yogurt (optional for extra creaminess and protein)

Ice cubes (optional)

Instructions:

- In a blender, combine mango, pineapple, banana, coconut water, and Greek yogurt (if using).
- Blend until smooth. Add ice to reach desired thickness, if needed.
- Serve immediately, garnished with a slice of pineapple or mango on the rim of the glass.

Nutritional Information (approximate per serving):

- Calories: 180
- Protein: 5g (with Greek yogurt)
- Fiber: 3g
- Calcium: 50mg (with Greek yogurt)

Peanut Butter Banana Oat Smoothie

Prep Time: 5 minutes

Cook Time: 0 minutes

Servings: 2

Ingredients:

2 bananas, sliced and frozen

2 tablespoons natural peanut butter

1/4 cup rolled oats

1 cup almond milk (fortified for additional nutrients)

1/2 teaspoon vanilla extract

Ice cubes (optional, for a thicker smoothie)

Optional: 1 tablespoon flaxseed meal (for omega-3s and fiber)

Instructions:

- Add bananas, peanut butter, oats, almond milk, vanilla extract, and flaxseed meal (if using) to a blender.
- Blend on high until smooth and creamy. Add ice if desired for thickness.
- Pour into glasses and serve for a filling and energizing smoothie.

Nutritional Information (approximate per serving):

Calories: 300

Protein: 8g

Fiber: 6g

Calcium: 150mg

Antioxidant Blueberry Almond Smoothie

Prep Time: 5 minutes

Cook Time: 0 minutes

Servings: 2

Ingredients:

- 1 cup blueberries, frozen
- 1 banana, sliced and frozen
- 1 cup spinach leaves (optional, for added nutrients)
- 1 cup almond milk (fortified to enhance calcium and vitamin D intake)
- 2 tablespoons almond butter (for healthy fats and protein)
- Optional: 1 teaspoon honey for sweetness

Instructions:

- In a blender, combine blueberries, banana, spinach (if using), almond milk, and almond butter.
- Blend until smooth. Sweeten with honey if desired.
- Serve immediately, enjoying the creamy texture and rich, antioxidant-packed flavors.

Nutritional Information (approximate per serving):

- Calories: 250
- Protein: 6g
- Fiber: 5g
- Calcium: 200mg

Super Seed and Fruit Smoothie

Prep Time: 5 minutes

Cook Time: 0 minutes

Servings: 2

Ingredients:

- 1 cup frozen mixed berries (strawberries, raspberries, blueberries)
- 1 ripe banana
- 1 tablespoon chia seeds
- 1 tablespoon hemp seeds
- 1 tablespoon flaxseed meal
- 1 cup spinach or kale (optional, for added nutrients)
- 1 1/2 cups oat milk (fortified, for added calcium and vitamins)
- Optional: A drizzle of honey or maple syrup for sweetness

Instructions:

- Place all ingredients in a blender, adding the leafy greens first if using.
- Blend on high until smooth and creamy. Add a bit of honey or maple syrup if extra sweetness is desired.
- Pour into glasses and serve immediately, garnished with a few whole berries or a sprinkle of seeds on top.

Nutritional Information (approximate per serving):

- Calories: 280
- Protein: 8g
- Fiber: 7g
- Calcium: 300mg

Refreshing Cucumber Mint Smoothie

Prep Time: 5 minutes

Cook Time: 0 minutes

Servings: 2

Ingredients:

- 1 large cucumber, peeled and chopped
- 1 cup plain Greek yogurt (for protein and calcium)
- Juice of 1 lime

- 1/4 cup fresh mint leaves
- 1/2 cup water or coconut water (for hydration)
- Ice cubes (optional, for a colder smoothie)
- Optional: 1 teaspoon honey for added sweetness

Instructions:

- Combine cucumber, Greek yogurt, lime juice, mint leaves, and water or coconut water in a blender. Add ice if using.
- Blend until smooth. Taste and add honey if desired for sweetness.
- Serve chilled, garnished with mint leaves or a slice of cucumber.

Nutritional Information (approximate per serving):

- Calories: 120
- Protein: 10g
- Fiber: 2g
- Calcium: 150mg

Carrot Cake Smoothie

Prep Time: 5 minutes

Cook Time: 0 minutes

Servings: 2

Ingredients:

- 1 cup carrot juice (for vitamin A and antioxidants)
- 1 ripe banana, frozen
- 1/4 cup rolled oats
- 1/2 teaspoon cinnamon
- 1/4 teaspoon nutmeg
- 1/2 cup plain Greek yogurt (for protein and calcium)
- 1 tablespoon walnuts (for omega-3 fatty acids)
- 1 tablespoon maple syrup (optional, for sweetness)
- Ice cubes (optional, for thickness)

Instructions:

- Add all ingredients to a blender, starting with the carrot juice to facilitate easier blending.
- Blend on high until smooth and creamy. Adjust sweetness with maple syrup if desired.
- Serve immediately, garnished with a sprinkle of cinnamon or a few walnut pieces.

Nutritional Information (approximate per serving):

- Calories: 220
- Protein: 8g

- Fiber: 3g

- Calcium: 150mg

Chocolate Avocado Smoothie

Prep Time: 5 minutes

Cook Time: 0 minutes

Servings: 2

Ingredients:

- 1 ripe avocado

- 2 tablespoons cocoa powder

- 1 1/2 cups almond milk (fortified, for added nutrients)

- 1 banana, frozen

- 1 tablespoon peanut butter (for protein and healthy fats)

- Optional: honey or maple syrup to taste

Instructions:

- Place avocado, cocoa powder, almond milk, banana, and peanut butter in a blender.

- Blend until smooth. Sweeten with honey or maple syrup if needed.

- Pour into glasses and serve immediately, perhaps with a dusting of cocoa powder on top.

Nutritional Information (approximate per serving):

- Calories: 300
- Protein: 6g
- Fiber: 9g
- Calcium: 200mg

Zesty Lemon Ginger Detox Smoothie

Prep Time: 5 minutes

Cook Time: 0 minutes

Servings: 2

Ingredients:

- 1 cup spinach or kale (for greens and vitamins)
- 1 apple, cored and sliced
- 1/2 cucumber, chopped
- Juice of 1 lemon
- 1 tablespoon fresh ginger, grated
- 1 cup water or coconut water (for hydration)
- Ice cubes (optional, for a chilled smoothie)

Instructions:

- Combine spinach or kale, apple, cucumber, lemon juice, ginger, and water or coconut water in a blender. Add ice if preferred.
- Blend on high until smooth and fully combined.
- Taste and adjust the lemon or ginger according to preference.
- Serve immediately, enjoying the refreshing and detoxifying benefits.

Nutritional Information (approximate per serving):

- Calories: 100
- Protein: 2g
- Fiber: 4g
- Calcium: 50mg

Quinoa Stuffed Bell Peppers

Prep Time: 15 minutes

Cook Time: 30 minutes

Servings: 4

Ingredients:

- 4 large bell peppers, tops cut off and seeds removed
- 1 cup quinoa, cooked
- 1 can (15 oz) black beans, rinsed and drained
- 1 cup corn kernels (fresh, canned, or thawed from frozen)
- 1/2 cup tomato sauce
- 1 teaspoon cumin
- 1 teaspoon paprika
- Salt and pepper to taste
- 1/2 cup shredded cheddar cheese (low-fat for calcium)
- Fresh cilantro for garnish

Instructions:

- Preheat oven to 375°F (190°C).

- In a bowl, mix the cooked quinoa, black beans, corn, tomato sauce, cumin, paprika, salt, and pepper.
- Stuff each bell pepper with the quinoa mixture and place in a baking dish.
- Cover with foil and bake for about 25 minutes. Uncover, top each pepper with cheese, and bake for an additional 5 minutes, or until the cheese is melted.
- Garnish with fresh cilantro before serving.

Nutritional Information (approximate per serving):

- Calories: 350
- Protein: 15g
- Fiber: 8g
- Calcium: 150mg

Lemon Herb Salmon

Prep Time: 10 minutes

Cook Time: 15 minutes

Servings: 4

Ingredients:

- 4 salmon fillets (6 oz each)
- 2 tablespoons olive oil

- Juice and zest of 1 lemon
- 2 garlic cloves, minced
- 1 tablespoon fresh dill, chopped
- 1 tablespoon fresh parsley, chopped
- Salt and pepper to taste
- Lemon slices for garnish

Instructions:

- Preheat the oven to 400°F (200°C). Line a baking sheet with parchment paper.
- In a small bowl, mix olive oil, lemon juice and zest, garlic, dill, and parsley. Season with salt and pepper.
- Place salmon fillets on the prepared baking sheet and brush each fillet with the lemon herb mixture.
- Bake for 12-15 minutes or until salmon flakes easily with a fork.
- Garnish with lemon slices and serve immediately.

Nutritional Information (approximate per serving):

- Calories: 300
- Protein: 23g
- Fiber: 0g
- Calcium: 30mg

Butternut Squash and Chickpea Curry

Prep Time: 15 minutes

Cook Time: 30 minutes

Servings: 4

Ingredients:

- 1 tablespoon coconut oil
- 1 onion, diced
- 2 cloves garlic, minced
- 1 tablespoon ginger, minced
- 1 butternut squash, peeled and cubed
- 1 can (15 oz) chickpeas, drained and rinsed
- 1 can (14 oz) coconut milk
- 2 teaspoons curry powder
- Salt and pepper to taste
- Fresh cilantro for garnish
- Cooked rice or naan for serving

Instructions:

- Heat coconut oil in a large skillet over medium heat. Add onion, garlic, and ginger, sautéing until onion is translucent.

- Add butternut squash, chickpeas, coconut milk, and curry powder. Season with salt and pepper.
- Bring to a boil, then reduce heat and simmer for 20-25 minutes, or until squash is tender.
- Serve over cooked rice or with naan, garnished with fresh cilantro.

Nutritional Information (approximate per serving, without rice/naan):

- Calories: 350
- Protein: 8g
- Fiber: 6g
- Calcium: 80mg

Garlic Parmesan Zucchini Noodles

Prep Time: 10 minutes

Cook Time: 10 minutes

Servings: 4

Ingredients:

- 4 zucchinis, spiralized
- 2 tablespoons olive oil
- 2 cloves garlic, minced

- Salt and pepper to taste
- 1/2 cup grated Parmesan cheese
- Red pepper flakes for garnish (optional)

Instructions:

- Heat olive oil in a large skillet over medium heat. Add minced garlic and sauté until fragrant.
- Add spiralized zucchini to the skillet. Season with salt and pepper, and cook for 5-7 minutes, or until noodles are tender.
- Remove from heat and stir in Parmesan cheese until melted and evenly distributed.
- Serve immediately, garnished with red pepper flakes if desired.

Nutritional Information (approximate per serving):

- Calories: 150
- Protein: 6g
- Fiber: 2g
- Calcium: 150mg

Chicken and Vegetable Stir-Fry

Prep Time: 15 minutes

Cook Time: 20 minutes

Servings: 4

Ingredients:

- 1 pound chicken breast, thinly sliced
- 2 tablespoons soy sauce (low sodium)
- 1 tablespoon sesame oil
- 1 cup broccoli florets
- 1 red bell pepper, sliced
- 1 carrot, julienned
- 2 cloves garlic, minced
- 1 tablespoon fresh ginger, minced
- 2 tablespoons oyster sauce
- 1 tablespoon honey
- Rice or noodles for serving

Instructions:

- Marinate chicken slices in soy sauce for at least 10 minutes.
- Heat sesame oil in a large skillet or wok over high heat. Add marinated chicken and stir-fry until cooked through. Remove chicken and set aside.
- In the same skillet, add broccoli, bell pepper, and carrot. Stir-fry for a few minutes until vegetables are tender but still crisp.

- Add garlic and ginger, cooking for another minute until fragrant.
- Return chicken to the skillet, add oyster sauce and honey, and stir well to combine.
- Serve hot over rice or noodles.

Nutritional Information (approximate per serving, without rice/noodles):

- Calories: 250
- Protein: 26g
- Fiber: 2g
- Calcium: 40mg

3 EXERCISE

Exercise and Lifestyle Changes for Bone Strength

Incorporating regular exercise and adopting specific lifestyle adjustments are essential techniques for boosting bone strength and general health. Let's study how combining particular types of physical activities and modifying daily routines may greatly contribute to bone density, minimize the risk of osteoporosis, and develop a healthy skeletal structure throughout life.

Exercise for Bone Health

1. **Weight-Bearing Exercises:** Activities that push you to work against gravity while standing upright are vital for bone health. Walking, jogging, hiking, and dancing come within this group. They aid in creating and maintaining bone density by activating bone-forming cells.

2. **Strength Training**: Utilizing weights or resistance bands not only develops muscular strength but also puts stress on bones, particularly in the hips, spine, and wrists, which are major sites

of fracture. Incorporating exercises like squats, lunges, and push-ups a few times a week can make a huge impact.

3. **Balance and Flexibility Workouts:** Practices such as yoga and tai chi enhance balance, coordination, and flexibility, lowering the risk of falls, especially in older persons. These workouts help strengthen the muscles that support bones, offering an added layer of protection.

4. **High-Impact Activities**: For people who can safely engage in high-impact workouts, activities like jogging, jump rope, or some forms of sports can further boost bone density. However, it's vital to build up to these activities gradually and evaluate any existing disorders that would make high-impact exercise inappropriate.

Lifestyle Changes for Stronger Bones

1. Nutrition: A balanced diet rich in calcium and vitamin D is vital. Calcium assists the formation and maintenance of bone structure, whereas vitamin D improves calcium absorption. meals such as dairy products, leafy green vegetables, fatty salmon, and fortified meals should be staples in your diet.

2. Sunshine Exposure: Regular, moderate exposure to sunshine helps the body generate vitamin D naturally. Depending on your region, skin type, and the time of year, even only 10-15 minutes of sun exposure several times a week can be helpful.

3. Moderation in Alcohol Consumption and Smoking: Both excessive drinking and smoking have been related to weakening bones and increased risk of osteoporosis. Reducing alcohol intake and stopping smoking can greatly enhance bone health and general well-being.

4. Monitoring Bone Health: Regular check-ups and bone density tests can help track bone health, especially if you have risk factors for osteoporosis. Early identification is crucial to controlling and minimizing bone health concerns.

5. Staying Hydrated: Adequate hydration is often forgotten in conversations about bone health. Water serves a key function in sustaining cellular health, particularly the cells that make our bones and the surrounding muscles.

Weight-bearing

Weight-bearing activities force you to work against gravity while standing, which helps to grow and maintain bone density. Here's a look at numerous workouts under this category, including how to execute them, recommended time allocation, and their benefits.

1. Walking

- **How to Do It**: Keep a quick pace, keep proper posture, and employ a complete heel-to-toe stride. Swing your arms naturally to enhance intensity.
- **Time Allocation**: Aim for at least 30 minutes on most days of the week. You may split this down into shorter, 10-minute walks if required.
- **Benefits**: Walking strengthens bones, especially in the legs and lower spine. It enhances cardiovascular health, muscular endurance, and balance, lowering the risk of osteoporosis and heart disease.

2. Stair Climbing

- **How to Do It**: Use the stairs instead of elevators when feasible. For a more planned workout, ascend and descend a set of steps repeatedly.
- **Time Allocation**: Start with 10 minutes if you're new to stair climbing, gradually increasing to 20-30 minutes as your stamina increases.
- **Benefits**: This workout targets your legs, hips, and lower spine, directly encouraging these bones to improve in

density. It also enhances cardiovascular health and leg strength.

3. Jump Rope

- **How to Do It**: Start with your feet slightly apart, gripping the rope handles alongside your torso. Swing the rope above your head and jump over it with both feet.
- **Time Allocation**: Begin with small periods of 30 seconds to 1 minute, aiming for a total of 10-15 minutes as you increase stamina.
- **Benefits**: Jumping rope is a high-impact workout that greatly builds bone density in the legs. It also promotes heart health, coordination, and balance.

4. Dancing

- **How to Do It**: Engage in whatever dancing style you prefer, whether it's ballroom, hip-hop, or ballet. Dance courses or home dance exercises both work.
- **Time Allocation**: Dance for at least 30 minutes to an hour for a thorough exercise that includes warm-up and cooldown periods.

- **Benefits**: Dancing is a joyful, full-body workout that increases bone density, flexibility, muscular strength, balance, and mental health.

5. Hiking

- **How to Do It**: Choose paths that match your fitness level, utilizing good hiking footwear for support. Challenge yourself with diverse terrains and inclines as you feel more comfortable.
- **Time Allocation**: Start with shorter trails that take roughly 30 minutes to finish, eventually building up to larger treks of 1-2 hours or more.
- **Benefits**: Hiking strengthens the bones in your legs and hips and promotes cardiovascular health. The varying terrain also promotes balance and stability.

6. Tennis or Badminton

- **How to Do It**: Engage in games of tennis or badminton, focusing on fast movements, hops, and dashes across the court.
- **Time Allocation**: Play for at least 30 minutes to an hour, depending on your fitness level and intensity of the game.

- **Benefits**: These activities give high-impact, multidirectional action that promotes bone density in the arms, legs, and spine. They also promote agility, coordination, and cardiovascular health.

General Tips for Weight-Bearing Exercises

- **Warm-Up**: Always start with a 5-10 minute warm-up to prepare your body for activity and lower the chance of injury.
- **Progress Gradually**: Increase the time and intensity of your exercises gradually to avoid overexertion and injury.
- **Mix It Up**: Incorporate a range of weight-bearing exercises throughout your regimen to activate different bone regions and keep workouts intriguing.
- **Stay Hydrated**: Drink lots of water before, during, and after exercise to stay hydrated.

Strength Training Exercise

Strength training, commonly known as resistance training, is vital for growing muscle mass and bone strength. By providing stress to the bones, these activities induce bone-forming cells to enhance bone density. Here's a closer look at strength training exercises, including how to practice them, suggested length, and their benefits to the body.

1. Chair Squats

- **How to Do It**: Starting Position: Place a chair behind you. Stand in front of the chair with your feet shoulder-width apart, toes pointing slightly outward. Keep your arms straight out in front of you, parallel to the floor, for balance.

- Initiate the Squat: Begin by softly bending at the hips and knees as if you are ready to sit down. Push your hips backward while maintaining your chest high and your back straight. Your weight should be on your heels, not your toes.

- Lower Down: Continue lowering yourself gently until your buttocks lightly contact the chair. Avoid totally sitting down or relaxing your muscles; instead, just touch the chair to check you're going low enough.

- Rising Up: Push through your heels to stand back up to the beginning posture. Keep your core engaged and keep a straight back as you ascend. Your arms can aid balance during the movement.

- Repeat: Perform 8-12 repetitions for 2-3 sets, resting for 1-2 minutes between sets. As you acquire strength, you may increase the amount of repetitions and sets.

- **Time Allocation**: Aim for 2-3 sets of 8-12 repetitions, resting for 1-2 minutes between sets.

- **Benefits**: Squats strengthen the bones and muscles of the lower body, especially the hips, thighs, and lower back. This exercise also improves balance and coordination, minimizing the risk of falls.

3. Wall Push-Ups

- **Starting Position:** Stand facing a wall, roughly an arm's length away. Place your palms flat against the wall at shoulder breadth and shoulder height.

- **Lower Your torso**: Keeping your feet grounded and torso straight, slowly bend your elbows to bring your chest nearer the wall. Your elbows should bend out to the sides.

- **Drive Back**: Press through your hands to drive your body back to the beginning position, straightening your arms.

- **Breathing**: Inhale as you lower your body towards the wall, and exhale as you push back to the starting position.

Time Allocation

- Frequency: Aim to do wall push-ups 2-3 times a week. This provides your muscles time to recuperate and strengthen between workouts.

- Duration: Start with 1 set of 8-12 repetitions. As your strength develops, steadily up to 2-3 sets.

- Rest: Rest for 1-2 minutes between sets to enable your muscles to recuperate.

Benefits to the Body for Seniors

- Upper Body Strength: Wall push-ups improve the chest, shoulders, and triceps, which are crucial for daily actions like opening doors, using a vacuum, or reaching for objects on a shelf.

- Improved Bone Health: This weight-bearing activity aids in maintaining bone density in the upper body, minimizing the incidence of osteoporosis.

- Enhanced Core Stability: Engaging the core during wall push-ups helps improve balance and posture, minimizing the chance of falls.

- Accessibility: Wall push-ups may be performed anyplace with a wall, making it a practical workout choice. They are also less scary than floor push-ups, promoting frequent activity.

- Joint-Friendly: For persons with wrist, elbow, or shoulder concerns, wall push-ups offer a low-impact option to strengthen these regions without undue strain.

Additional Tips

- **Keep the Core Engaged**: Tighten your abdominal muscles during the workout to support your back and increase stability.

- **Progress Gradually**: As you get more comfortable and stronger, you may raise the intensity by standing further from the wall or shifting to more strenuous versions like incline push-ups on a solid bench.

- **Listen to Your Body**: If you encounter any pain or discomfort, alter your form or speak with a physical therapist to verify you're executing the exercise correctly.

General Tips for Strength Training Form First:

- Prioritize perfect form to maximize benefits and limit the chance of injury.

- Consistency: Incorporate strength training into your regimen 2-3 times per week, allowing for rest days in between to enable muscles recuperate.

- Progressive Overload: Gradually increase the weight or resistance as your strength develops to continue testing your bones and muscles.

- Balanced Diet: Support your exercise with a nutrient-rich diet high in calcium, vitamin D, and protein to help in bone and muscle development.

- Strength training is a strong strategy for boosting bone density and general physical health. It's useful for persons of all ages, especially those at risk for those dealing with osteoporosis.

Balance and flexibility exercises

Balance and flexibility exercises are vital components of a well-rounded fitness plan, especially for seniors. Improving balance can greatly lower the chance of falls, a key issue for older persons, while boosting flexibility adds to a broader range of motion, reduced muscular stiffness, and decreased risk of injuries. Here's how seniors may add balance and flexibility exercises into their routines:

Balance Exercises for Seniors 1. Single-Leg Stance

- **How to Do It:** Stand behind a strong chair, holding on for support. Lift one foot off the floor, retaining the position for as long as comfortable. Switch legs and repeat.

- **Time Allocation**: Aim for 10-30 seconds each leg, repeating 2-3 times.

- **Benefits:** Strengthens leg muscles and improves general stability.

2. Heel-to-Toe Walk

- **How to Do It**: Place the heel of one foot directly in front of the toes of the opposing foot each time you take a stride. Your heel and toes should touch or almost touch. Extend your arms outward to maintain balance.

- **Time Allocation**: Walk 15-20 steps this manner, 1-2 times per session.

- **Benefits**: Enhances coordination and balance, simulating ordinary motions.

Flexibility Exercises for Seniors

1. Seated Forward Bend

- **How to Do It**: Sit on the edge of a chair with your legs out in front of you. Hinge at the hips and bend forward, reaching towards your toes. Hold when you feel a stretch in your hamstrings.
- **Time Allocation**: Hold for 15-30 seconds, repeating 2-3 times.
- **Benefits**: Increases flexibility in the hamstrings and lower back, improving improved posture and minimizing lower back stiffness.

2. Upper Body Stretch

- **How to Do It:** Sit or stand erect. Reach your arms overhead, clasping your hands together. Gently lean to one side until you feel a stretch down your side. Return to center and lean to the opposite side.
- **Time Allocation**: Hold each side for 15-30 seconds, repeating 2-3 times.
- **Benefits**: Improves flexibility in the shoulders, arms, and sides of the body, assisting in daily activities that involve reaching or bending.

General Tips for Balance and Flexibility Training

- Warm-Up: Start with a mild warm-up to get the blood flowing and prepare your muscles for stretching, such as walking or marching in place for a few minutes.

- Consistency: Practice balance and flexibility exercises frequently, aiming for most days of the week. Consistency is crucial to witnessing progress.

- Breathe: Remember to breathe regularly during these workouts. Holding your breath can cause tension in your muscles.

- Listen to Your Body: Stretch to the point of moderate discomfort, not agony. If a workout causes discomfort, stop and talk with a healthcare practitioner.

- Use Support When Needed: For balancing exercises, have a chair or wall nearby for support if you feel unstable.

Reducing Risk Factors for Osteoporosis

Reducing risk factors for osteoporosis is critical, especially for seniors, since it directly effects their quality of life and independence. Osteoporosis, characterized by weaker bones that are more vulnerable to fractures, can be strongly impacted by lifestyle choices and environmental variables. Here are techniques to lessen the risk:

1. **Adequate Calcium Intake Strategy**: Ensure a diet rich in calcium, which is crucial for bone health. Seniors should aim for roughly 1,200 mg of calcium per day, which may be reached through both food sources and supplementation if necessary.

Sources: Dairy products (milk, yogurt, cheese), leafy green vegetables (kale, broccoli), fortified meals (cereals, orange juice), and almonds.

2. **Sufficient Vitamin D Strategy**: Vitamin D is necessary for calcium absorption. Seniors require 800 to 1,000 IU of vitamin D daily, which can come from sunshine, food, and supplementation.

Sources: Fatty fish (salmon, mackerel), egg yolks, fortified meals, and sunshine exposure. Just 10-15 minutes of sun exposure a few times a week will assist, although this varies depends on geographic area, skin type, and season.

3. **Regular Exercise Strategy**: Engage in regular weight-bearing and muscle-strengthening activities to enhance bone density and strength. Balance exercises are also vital to lower the risk of falls.

Types: Walking, stair climbing, tai chi, yoga, and resistance activities like lifting weights or utilizing resistance bands.

4. **Avoid Smoking and Limit Alcohol Intake Strategy**: Smoking and excessive alcohol use are associated to increased bone loss and risk of fractures. Quitting smoking and restricting drinking to reasonable amounts are key preventative strategies.

Implementation: Seek help for smoking cessation and limit alcohol intake to suggested levels (up to one drink a day for women and two for men).

5. **Fall Prevention Strategy:** Implement home safety measures to limit the chance of falls, which can lead to fractures. This involves reducing trip hazards, enhancing lighting, and adding grab bars in crucial locations like the restroom.

Implementation: Regularly examine the living environment for dangers and consider the use of assistive equipment like walkers or canes if balance is an issue.

6. **Medication Review Strategy**: Some drugs may lead to bone loss or increase the risk of falls. Regularly examine all drugs with a healthcare provider.

Implementation: Discuss with doctors the potential of altering drugs that can influence bone density or balance.

7. **Monitor Bone Health Strategy**: Regular bone density testing can help diagnose osteoporosis early, allowing for prompt action to limit development.

Implementation: Follow healthcare providers' recommendations for bone density examinations, especially if you have risk factors for osteoporosis.

8. **Healthy Weight Maintenance Strategy**: Being underweight might raise the risk of bone loss and fractures. Maintaining a healthy weight is vital for bone health.

Implementation: Balanced nutrition and regular exercise can assist reach and maintain a healthy weight.

FOUR WEEKS MEAL PLAN

Day	Breakfast	Snack	Dinner	Dessert
1	Spinach Avocado Green Smoothie	Greek Yogurt and Berry Parfait	Quinoa Stuffed Bell Peppers	Avocado Chocolate Mousse
2	Berry Blast Protein Smoothie	Almond and Date Energy Balls	Lemon Herb Salmon with steamed broccoli	Baked Apple Slices with Cinnamon
3	Tropical Mango Pineapple Smoothie	Avocado Toast with Pumpkin Seeds	Butternut Squash and Chickpea Curry with brown rice	No-Bake Peanut Butter Oat Bars
4	Peanut Butter Banana Oat Smoothie	Cottage Cheese and Fruit Bowl	Garlic Parmesan Zucchini Noodles	Mixed Berry Yogurt Parfait
5	Antioxidant Blueberry Almond Smoothie	Veggie Sticks with Hummus	Chicken and Vegetable Stir-Fry with quinoa	Coconut Rice Pudding
6	Oatmeal with Fresh Berries	Baked Sweet Potato Chips	Roasted Eggplant and Tomato Pasta	Lemon Chia Seed Pudding
7	Whole Wheat Toast with Avocado and	Roasted Chickpeas	Lemon Garlic Shrimp and Asparagus with side salad	Frozen Yogurt Bark with Mixed Berries

scrambled
eggs

WEEK TWO MEAL PLAN

Day	Breakfast	Lunch	Dinner	Snack	Dessert
1	Spinach Avocado Green Smoothie	Tomato Basil Soup with Whole Grain Bread	Quinoa Stuffed Bell Peppers	Greek Yogurt and Berry Parfait	Avocado Chocolate Mousse
2	Berry Blast Protein Smoothie	Veggie Hummus Wrap	Lemon Herb Salmon with Steamed Broccoli	Almond and Date Energy Balls	Baked Apple Slices with Cinnamon
3	Tropical Mango Pineapple Smoothie	Quinoa and Black Bean Bowl	Butternut Squash and Chickpea Curry with Brown Rice	Avocado Toast with Pumpkin Seeds	No-Bake Peanut Butter Oat Bars
4	Peanut Butter Banana Oat Smoothie	Tuna Salad Stuffed Avocado	Garlic Parmesan Zucchini Noodles	Cottage Cheese and Fruit Bowl	Mixed Berry Yogurt Parfait
5	Oatmeal	Grilled	Chicken	Baked	Coconut

Day	Breakfast	Lunch	Dinner	Snack	Dessert
	with Fresh Berries	Chicken Salad	and Vegetable Stir-Fry with Quinoa	Sweet Potato Chips	Rice Pudding
6	Whole Wheat Toast with Avocado and Scrambled Eggs	Egg Salad on Whole Grain Toast	Roasted Eggplant and Tomato Pasta	Roasted Chickpeas	Lemon Chia Seed Pudding
7	Antioxidant Blueberry Almond Smoothie	Cottage Cheese with Pineapple and Walnuts	Lemon Garlic Shrimp and Asparagus with Side Salad	Veggie Sticks with Hummus	Frozen Yogurt Bark with Mixed Berries

WEEK THREE MEAL PLAN

Day	Breakfast	Lunch	Dinner	Snack	Dessert
1	Oatmeal with Fresh Berries	Egg Salad on Whole Grain Toast	Lemon Garlic Shrimp and Asparagus	Greek Yogurt and Berry Parfait	Baked Apple Slices with Cinnamon
2	Peanut Butter Banana	Tomato Basil Soup	Garlic Parmesan	Cottage Cheese and Fruit	Lemon Chia Seed Pudding

	Oat Smoothie	with Whole Grain Bread	Zucchini Noodles	Bowl	
3	Antioxidant Blueberry Almond Smoothie	Quinoa and Black Bean Bowl	Chicken and Vegetable Stir-Fry with Quinoa	Avocado Toast with Pumpkin Seeds	Avocado Chocolate Mousse
4	Tropical Mango Pineapple Smoothie	Grilled Chicken Salad	Roasted Eggplant and Tomato Pasta	Veggie Sticks with Hummus	No-Bake Peanut Butter Oat Bars
5	Spinach Avocado Green Smoothie	Veggie Hummus Wrap	Butternut Squash and Chickpea Curry with Brown Rice	Almond and Date Energy Balls	Mixed Berry Yogurt Parfait
6	Berry Blast Protein Smoothie	Tuna Salad Stuffed Avocado	Quinoa Stuffed Bell Peppers	Baked Sweet Potato Chips	Coconut Rice Pudding
7	Whole Wheat Toast with Avocado and Scrambled Eggs	Cottage Cheese with Pineapple and Walnuts	Lemon Herb Salmon with Steamed Broccoli	Roasted Chickpeas	Frozen Yogurt Bark with Mixed Berries

WEEK FOUR MEAL PLAN

Day	Breakfast	Lunch	Dinner	Snack	Dessert
1	Spinach Avocado Green Smoothie	Quinoa and Black Bean Bowl	Lemon Garlic Shrimp and Asparagus	Roasted Chickpeas	Coconut Rice Pudding
2	Berry Blast Protein Smoothie	Tomato Basil Soup with Whole Grain Bread	Quinoa Stuffed Bell Peppers	Greek Yogurt and Berry Parfait	Lemon Chia Seed Pudding
3	Peanut Butter Banana Oat Smoothie	Egg Salad on Whole Grain Toast	Garlic Parmesan Zucchini Noodles	Cottage Cheese and Fruit Bowl	Baked Apple Slices with Cinnamon
4	Oatmeal with Fresh Berries	Grilled Chicken Salad	Chicken and Vegetable Stir-Fry with Quinoa	Veggie Sticks with Hummus	Avocado Chocolate Mousse
5	Tropical Mango Pineapple Smoothie	Veggie Hummus Wrap	Roasted Eggplant and Tomato	Almond and Date Energy	No-Bake Peanut Butter

			Pasta	Balls	Oat Bars
6	Whole Wheat Toast with Avocado and Scrambled Eggs	Tuna Salad Stuffed Avocado	Butternut Squash and Chickpea Curry with Brown Rice	Baked Sweet Potato Chips	Mixed Berry Yogurt Parfait
7	Antioxidant Blueberry Almond Smoothie	Cottage Cheese with Pineapple and Walnuts	Lemon Herb Salmon with Steamed Broccoli	Avocado Toast with Pumpkin Seeds	Frozen Yogurt Bark with Mixed Berries

Weekly Exercise Schedule Plan

Day 1: Strength Training

- **Activity**: Upper body strength training
- **Details**: Perform exercises like wall push-ups, seated bicep curls, and shoulder presses using light weights or resistance bands.
- **Duration**: 30 minutes

Day 2: Cardiovascular Exercise

- **Activity**: Walking or Aqua Aerobics

- **Details**: Choose a brisk walk outdoors or participate in an aqua aerobics class if you have access to a pool.
- **Duration**: 30-45 minutes

Day 3: Flexibility and Balance

- **Activity**: Yoga or Tai Chi
- **Details**: Attend a gentle yoga class or follow a tai chi video designed for seniors, focusing on balance and flexibility.
- **Duration**: 30-45 minutes

Day 4: Rest or Gentle Activity

- **Activity**: Rest or gentle stretching
- **Details**: Take a complete rest day or engage in gentle stretching exercises to keep the muscles limber without strain.
- **Duration**: 15-20 minutes of stretching, if chosen

Day 5: Strength Training

- **Activity**: Lower body strength training
- **Details**: Focus on exercises like seated leg lifts, chair squats, and calf raises to strengthen the lower body.
- **Duration**: 30 minutes

Day 6: Cardiovascular Exercise

- **Activity**: Cycling or Swimming
- **Details**: Go for a gentle bike ride or swim laps at a comfortable pace, focusing on steady, low-impact movement.
- **Duration**: 30-45 minutes

Day 7: Balance and Flexibility

- **Activity**: Pilates or Balance Exercises
- **Details**: Engage in a Pilates session focusing on core strength and flexibility, or practice balance exercises like the single-leg stand.
- **Duration**: 30-45 minutes

CONVERSION CHART

Measurement	Equivalent
Volume	
1 tablespoon (tbsp)	3 teaspoons (tsp)
1 cup	16 tablespoons (tbsp)
1 cup	8 fluid ounces (fl oz)
1 pint (pt)	2 cups
1 quart (qt)	2 pints (pt)
1 gallon (gal)	4 quarts (qt)
Weight	
1 ounce (oz)	28.35 grams (g)
1 pound (lb)	16 ounces (oz)
1 kilogram (kg)	2.20462 pounds (lb)
Length	
1 inch (in)	2.54 centimeters (cm)
1 foot (ft)	12 inches (in)
1 yard (yd)	3 feet (ft)
1 meter (m)	3.28084 feet (ft)
Temperature	
32°F	0°C (freezing point of water)
212°F	100°C (boiling point of water)
350°F	177°C (common baking temperature)

Grocery List

Fruits and Vegetables

Avocados

Spinach

Mangoes

Pineapples

Berries (strawberries, blueberries, raspberries)

Fresh herbs (basil, parsley, cilantro, dill)

Asparagus

Butternut squash

Cucumbers

Potatoes (for baking)

Apples

Chicken breasts or thighs

Garlic

Lemons and limes

Tomatoes and cherry tomatoes

Bell peppers (various colors)

Eggplants

Zucchini

Broccoli

Carrots

Mixed greens for salads

Onions

Proteins

Salmon fillets

Shrimp

Canned tuna

Eggs

Canned chickpeas

Cottage cheese

Greek yogurt (plain)

Canned black beans

Grains and Cereals

Quinoa

Whole grain or whole wheat bread

Brown rice

Whole grain wraps

Oatmeal

Dairy and Alternatives

Milk (or plant-based alternatives like almond milk, oat milk)

Feta cheese

Parmesan cheese

Nuts, Seeds, and Legumes

Almonds

Walnuts

Pumpkin seeds

Chia seeds

Date

Peanut butter (natural)

Pantry Staples

Olive oil

Sesame oil

Balsamic vinegar or other vinaigrettes

Tomato sauce and tomato soup

Honey or maple syrup

Dark chocolate chips

Coconut milk

Canned tomatoes

Vegetable or chicken broth

Soy sauce (low sodium)

Spices (cumin, paprika, curry powder, cinnamon, nutmeg, salt, pepper)

Snacks

Hummus

Sweet potatoes (for chips)

Coconut oil

Whole grain or multigrain crackers

Freezer Items

Frozen berries (if fresh are not available or for smoothies)

Frozen mixed vegetables (for stir-fries)

Baking and Cooking Essentials

Flour (for any baking needs)

Baking powder and baking soda (if needed)

Vanilla extra

CONCLUSION

We appreciate your effort in exploring " OSTEOPOROSIS DIET COOKBOOK FOR SENIORS Through Diet and Lifestyle." This book serves as both a collection of essential information and an exploration of the quiet yet serious health issue of osteoporosis, offering insights and strategies for conquering it.

Within the contents of this text, we have explored the significant impact that nutrition and lifestyle have on the management and potential reversal of osteoporosis. The tactics included in this guide, including nutrient-rich foods and individualized workout routines, are intended to empower you, the reader, to take control of your bone health.

Important Observations:

Osteoporosis is not an unavoidable aspect of the aging process; there are efficacious methods to improve bone health through proactive efforts.

The interplay between nutrition and exercise has a crucial role in both preventing and managing osteoporosis.

Comprehending the specific requirements of your own body and making necessary adjustments to your lifestyle is essential for efficient treatment.

Dear readers, I urge you to wholeheartedly adopt the concepts presented in this book, not as temporary solutions, but as enduring and ingrained habits for life. Interact with healthcare professionals to customize these suggestions according to your own health profiles. Remember, every step taken is a step toward stronger bones and a healthy life.

Finally, I urge you to share the information you've received. Discuss it with friends, family, or anybody who could benefit. Spreading awareness and developing understanding are just as vital as adopting these behaviors yourself.

Thank you once again for joining me on this crucial trip. Here's to a healthy, stronger future, free from the confines of osteoporosis. Let's continue to learn, progress, and encourage one other. Your journey to a vigorous life, replete with vitality and power, begins now.

Meal planner

DAYS	BREAKFAST	LUNCH	DINNER
MON			
TUE			
WED			
THU			
FRI			
SAT			
SUN			

GROSIRIES

-
-
-
-

NOTES

Meal planner

DAYS	BREAKFAST	LUNCH	DINNER
MON			
TUE			
WED			
THU			
FRI			
SAT			
SUN			

GROSIRIES

- ____
- ____
- ____
- ____

NOTES

Meal planner

DAYS	BREAKFAST	LUNCH	DINNER
MON			
TUE			
WED			
THU			
FRI			
SAT			
SUN			

GROSIRIES

-
-
-
-

NOTES

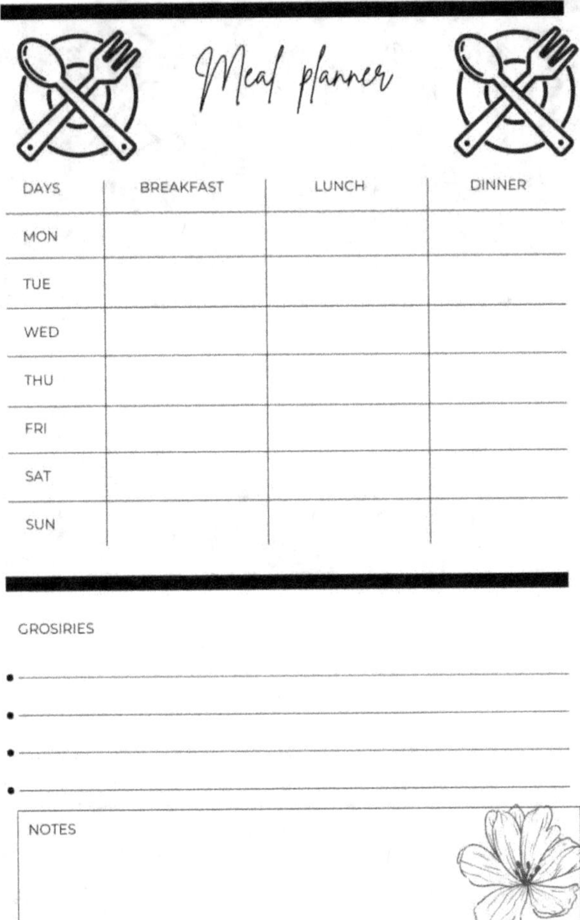

Meal planner

DAYS | BREAKFAST | LUNCH | DINNER
MON
TUE
WED
THU
FRI
SAT
SUN

GROSIRIES

NOTES

Meal planner

DAYS	BREAKFAST	LUNCH	DINNER
MON			
TUE			
WED			
THU			
FRI			
SAT			
SUN			

GROSIRIES

-
-
-
-

NOTES

Meal planner

DAYS	BREAKFAST	LUNCH	DINNER
MON			
TUE			
WED			
THU			
FRI			
SAT			
SUN			

GROSIRIES

- _______________________________________
- _______________________________________
- _______________________________________
- _______________________________________

NOTES

Meal planner

DAYS	BREAKFAST	LUNCH	DINNER
MON			
TUE			
WED			
THU			
FRI			
SAT			
SUN			

GROSIRIES

-
-
-
-

NOTES

$$Meal\ planner$$

DAYS	BREAKFAST	LUNCH	DINNER
MON			
TUE			
WED			
THU			
FRI			
SAT			
SUN			

GROSIRIES

- ____
- ____
- ____
- ____

NOTES

Meal planner

DAYS	BREAKFAST	LUNCH	DINNER
MON			
TUE			
WED			
THU			
FRI			
SAT			
SUN			

GROSIRIES

-
-
-
-

NOTES

Meal planner

DAYS	BREAKFAST	LUNCH	DINNER
MON			
TUE			
WED			
THU			
FRI			
SAT			
SUN			

GROSIRIES

- ____________________
- ____________________
- ____________________
- ____________________

NOTES

Meal planner

DAYS	BREAKFAST	LUNCH	DINNER
MON			
TUE			
WED			
THU			
FRI			
SAT			
SUN			

GROSIRIES

-
-
-
-

NOTES

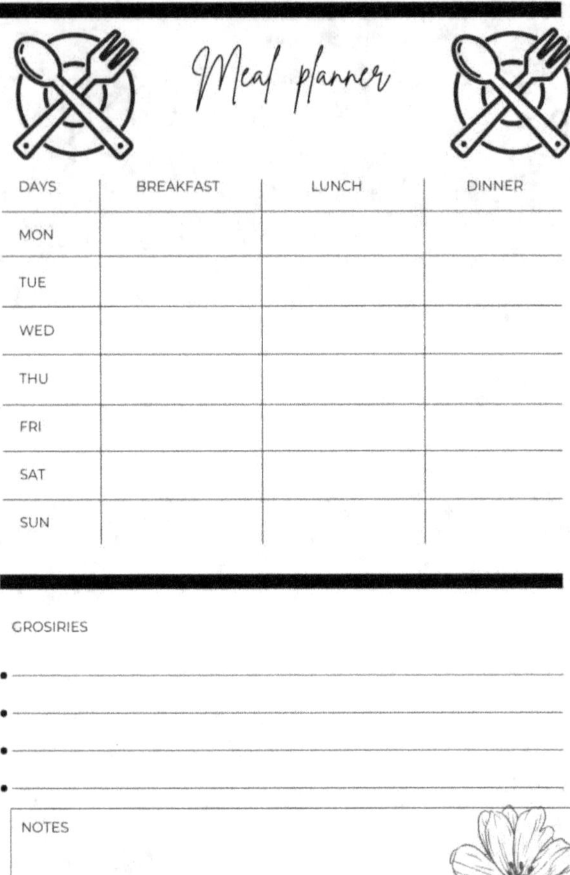

Meal planner
DAYS | BREAKFAST | LUNCH | DINNER
MON
TUE
WED
THU
FRI
SAT
SUN
GROSIRIES
NOTES

Meal planner

DAYS	BREAKFAST	LUNCH	DINNER
MON			
TUE			
WED			
THU			
FRI			
SAT			
SUN			

GROSIRIES

-
-
-
-

NOTES

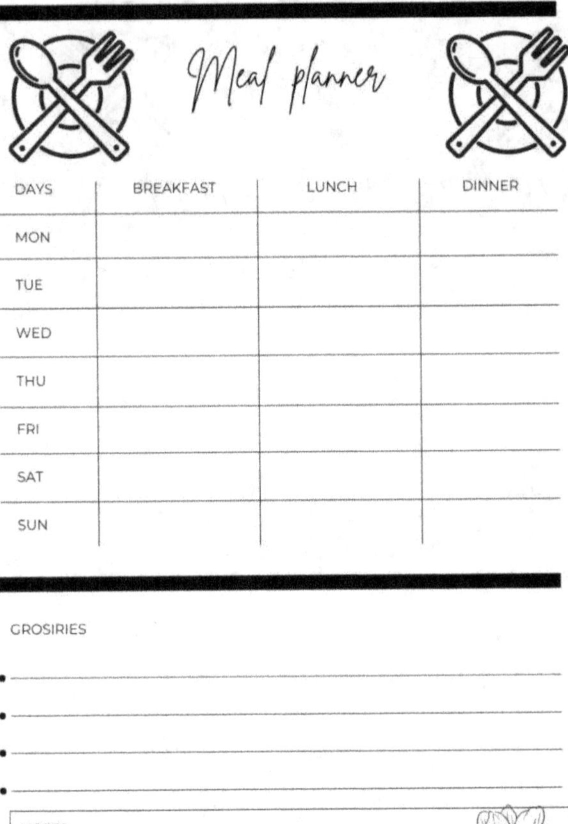

Meal planner
DAYS
BREAKFAST
LUNCH
DINNER
MON
TUE
WED
THU
FRI
SAT
SUN
GROSIRIES
NOTES